Life of
Christian Samuel
HAHNEMANN
Founder of Homœopathy

By
ROSA WAUGH HOBHOUSE

Author of
Life of Benjamin Waugh, The Divine Art of Healing, etc.

With a Preface by
SIR JOHN WEIR, K.C.V.O., M.B.

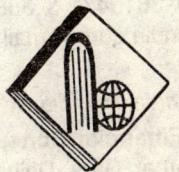

B. Jain Publishers Pvt. Ltd.
Delhi

> **NOTE FROM THE PUBLISHERS**
> Any information given in this book is not intended to be taken as a replacement for medical advice. Any person with a condition requiring medical attention should consult a qualified practitioner or therapist.

© All rights are reserved. No part of this publication may be reproduced, stored in a retrieval system or transmitted, in any form or by any means, mechanical, photocopying, recording or otherwise, without prior written permission of the publishers.

Price: Rs. 90.00

Reprint Edition: 2001 | 2002

Published by

KULDEEP JAIN

for

B. Jain Publishers (P) Ltd.

1921, Chuna Mandi, St. 10th, Paharganj,
New Delhi-110 055
Ph: 3670430, 3670572, 3683200, 3683300
Fax: 011-3610471 & 3683400
Website: www.bjainindia.com, Email: bjain@vsnl.com

Printed in India by
Unisons Techno Financial Consultants (P) Ltd.
522, FIE, Patpar Ganj, Delhi-110 092

ISBN 81-7021-685-0
BOOK CODE B-2283

PREFACE

It is difficult, even now, to estimate the influence on medicine of Samuel Hahnemann, whose "glorious discontent" with the therapeutics of his day was such that he gave up everything in the endeavour to find "if God had not indeed given some certain law by which the diseases of mankind could be cured." And to this patient genius the Law of Healing in time revealed itself, and to the elucidation of that Law he thereafter devoted his long life.

Hahnemann looked for his vindication to posterity. He envisaged the long years wherein some of the essentials among his "doctrines" would be questioned even by his own followers. But now, at last, his dicta are appealing to the more independent thinkers in medicine, although the limits of his teachings and suggestions are by no means reached, even in our day of scientific research. Hahnemann has always been, not only up-to-date, but before-date; and this still obtains.

It was long ago acknowledged by one of the pioneers of vaccine therapy that this practice was homœopathic; but it is only when such remedies are used, after the modified methods of Hahnemann, that the best results are obtained.

And now, in addition to vaccines, modern science is experimenting with another group of agents, homœopathically applied, for the cure of asthma, hay fever and other diseases of foreign protein origin. Homœopathic remedies are derived from all nature, since Hahnemann laid it down that any agent with power to adversely affect life—health—sensation—function—and, especially, mind—can be used for curative purposes. Power to hurt implies power to heal; these are but different degrees of the same thing: as is proved also by the Arndt-Schultz Law, "that the same substance which in large doses will prove lethal, and in smaller doses inhibitive, will, in minimal doses, prove stimulative to the same cells." Hence, even from the standpoint of modern science, Hahnemann's extensive and painstaking provings are more than justified!

Hahnemann recognised that drugging must always be worse than useless, because cure can only come by the stimulation of vital reactions against the "morbific" forces of disease. Here again modern science is demonstrating that he was correct in his contention, that curative remedies do not act directly on the tissues, but that, by stimulating the already existing vital reactions of the patient, they cause him to cure himself. Many of our leading pharmacologists are coming to believe in the indirect, rather than the direct action of drugs—to realise that it is in the complex life mechanisms of the sick person that the restoration to health must be looked for: that the *patient* is the *important* factor in the fight with disease.

Thus steadily, year by year, Hahnemann is coming into his own, and readers of this book will be enlightened by Mrs. Hobhouse's simple and enthusiastic setting forth of the life of this great pioneer; and we are indeed grateful to her for her self-imposed and arduous task.

6th May, 1933.   JOHN WEIR.

AUTHOR'S FOREWORD

My indebtedness to the late Dr. Richard Haehl of Stuttgart, author of *Samuel Hahnemann: His Life and Work*, and to his English translators will be apparent to all who know the two large volumes of this comprehensive work.

I am also indebted to my husband, Stephen Hobhouse, who in the autumn of 1931 visited Meissen, Köthen, and other places in Germany associated with Hahnemann's life, and by whose German scholarship I have been greatly helped. Besides having utilised passages from his letters giving local colour, my subject matter has been substantially increased by his efforts. In these Stephen Hobhouse was generously assisted by Dr. phil. Erich Preuss, at that time in Meissen, to whom my gratitude is also due. A promise of personal co-operation had been received from Dr. Richard Haehl, but his untimely death robbed us of the opportunity of availing ourselves of this privilege.

Thanks to Mrs. Marie Wheeler, it has been possible to consult a copy of the German original of Dr. Haehl's admirable biography; also for permission to use a number of the illustrations of both editions I have to express my gratitude to Mr. Mazzini Stuart and to Dr. Willmar Schwabe of Leipzig, to whom the blocks belong.

To Dr. Tyler, Editor of *Homœopathy*, who has spared for me some of her much-claimed time, thanks are again due.

The work has also been facilitated by my freedom as a member of the "British Homœopathic Association" to obtain books, such as Bradford's *Life and Letters of Dr. Samuel Hahnemann*, from the Tate Library, Chalmers House, 43 Russell Square, W.C.1.

A further acknowledgement of invaluable assistance must be given to C. E. Wheeler, M.D., B.S., B.Sc., who has kindly checked the work on its medical side. Indeed, it was largely due to this promise of oversight that I found courage to embark on so important a task as the presentation to the English public of Christian Samuel Hahnemann and his contribution to the science and art of healing.

ROSA WAUGH HOBHOUSE
Broxbourne,
May, 1933.

CONTENTS

PREFACE 5
By Sir John Weir, K.C.V.O., M.B.

FOREWORD 7

CHAPTER I

THE MEISSEN PORCELAIN PAINTERS 13
Meissen, 1755-1770

CHAPTER II

STUDENTSHIP AND QUALIFICATION 27
Meissen, Leipzig, Vienna, Hermannstadt, Erlangen, 1770-1779

CHAPTER III

FIRST PRACTICE AND MARRIAGE .. 47
Hettstedt, Dessau, Gommern, Dresden, Leipzig, 1779-1789

CHAPTER IV

POVERTY AND GROWING RECOGNITION 67
Leipzig, 1789-1792

CHAPTER V

HAHNEMANN AS PHYSICIAN OF THE MENTALLY DISORDERED
Georgenthal, 1792-1793

85

CHAPTER VI

THE APOTHECARIES' LEXICON AND THE FRIEND OF HEALTH —PART II
Molschleben, Göttingen, Pyrmont, Wolfenbüttel, Brunswick, 1793-1796

10

CHAPTER VII

THE NEW PRINCIPLE DECLARED
Königslutter, near Brunswick, 1796-1799

121

CHAPTER VIII

THE HIPPOCRATES OF THE INFINITELY LITTLE
Years covered by Chapters VII and IX

139

CHAPTER IX

"ÆSCULAPIUS IN THE BALANCE"
Hamburg-Altona, Mölln, Machern, Eilenburg, Dessau, Torgau, 1799-1811

155

CHAPTER X

HAHNEMANN AND HIS CIRCLE
Leipzig, 1811-1820

173

CONTENTS

CHAPTER XI

THE LEIPZIG APOTHECARIES .. 195
Leipzig and Köthen, 1820-1821

CHAPTER XII

HAHNEMANN AS COURT PHYSICIAN 215
Köthen, 1821-1830

CHAPTER XIII

INTERNATIONAL DEVELOPMENTS 237
Köthen, 1830-1832

CHAPTER XIV

SECOND MARRIAGE AND CLOSING DAYS IN PARIS 253
Paris, 1832-1843

BIBLIOGRAPHY 277

INDEX 283

[For List of Illustrations see over.]

LIST OF ILLUSTRATIONS

BUST OF HAHNEMANN BY WOLTRECK	*Frontispiece*
	Facing page
THE HOUSE WHERE HAHNEMANN WAS BORN	16
IVORY FAN PAINTED BY HAHNEMANN'S FATHER	17
LEIPZIG UNIVERSITY IN HAHNEMANN'S TIME	32
HAHNEMANN'S 'REBUS'	33
HAHNEMANN, FROM AN ETCHING	144
HAHNEMANN'S DAUGHTER, CHARLOTTE	145
HENRIETTE, HAHNEMANN'S WIFE	160
DR. JOHANN ERNST STAPF	161
FERDINAND, DUKE OF ANHALT-KÖTHEN	208
DR. GOTTFRIED LEHMANN	209
CERTIFICATE FROM LEIPZIG UNIVERSITY	210
DUCAL PATENT AS HOFRAT	220
MEDIZINALRAT DR. K. J. AEGIDI	224
CENTRAL FIGURE OF THE HAHNEMANN MEMORIAL IN WASHINGTON, U.S.A.	225
HAHNEMANN IN 1835	262
MADAME MELANIE, HAHNEMANN'S SECOND WIFE	263
PAGE OF HAHNEMANN'S HANDWRITING	270

Life of Christian Samuel Hahnemann

CHAPTER I

THE MEISSEN PORCELAIN PAINTERS

Meissen, 1755-1770

To the traveller who has been moving across the illimitable plains of Prussia it is a welcome change to come at last, in the neighbourhood of the Saxon town of Meissen, to the first low hills which herald the highlands that border the frontiers of South-West Germany. Here the broad Elbe is flowing between heights planted with forest trees and sometimes with the vine. The ancient town in recent years celebrated the thousandth anniversary of its birth, and prides itself on its magnificently situated castle and cathedral of mediæval memories, the Albrechtsburg and the Albrechtsdom.

Apart from its modern outgrowth on the northern bank of the Elbe, the main features of Meissen are still much as they were in Samuel Hahnemann's youthful days, which fell about the middle of the eighteenth century. The houses are crowded along the base and slopes of a long and beautiful valley running back from the main river. One side of this is still wooded, while the other is dominated by the cathedral and castle. Next to this the extensive buildings of St. Afra's are conspicuous, the Prince's or Fürsten-Schule, where Hahnemann studied as a boy. From the Freiheit, the "Liberty" of this school where the masters live, one looks down upon a picturesque mass of high, gabled roofs running down to the market and the beautiful "Frauenkirche," the church to which the Hahnemann family belonged. These still form, as in his time, the central feature of the higher portion of the little town.

In the neighbourhood of Meissen the clay soil in times past proved itself to be especially serviceable for the making of porcelain. Otherwise it is probable that Meissen would never have been associated with perfection in the art of porcelain making, and the beautiful china which it produces. Incidentally, it was due to this fact that the name of this Saxon town is also bound up with a vital episode in the history of the science and art of medicine. This was as the birthplace of Christian Samuel Hahnemann, who has in recent years been described by a living physician as "one of the great geniuses and patient investigators of the world"—one who pleaded that the *Materia Medica* of the profession should be "the pure reply of Nature to careful questioning." In his untiring experiments and clinical observations (recorded as indefatigably as they were prosecuted), he anticipated the methods of that "active army of investigators" of whom Raphael

THE MEISSEN PAINTERS

Meldola speaks in his introduction to *Chemistry*, who, in modern times, are devoting themselves to the study of Nature at first hand, and have become aware of the supreme importance of their work to the future welfare of the race. It is with this eighteenth-century German doctor and chemist, and those who assisted him in his life work of medical research, that our present biography is concerned.

The establishment of a porcelain factory at Meissen was, primarily, due not so much to the presence of the necessary raw material in the neighbourhood as to the then Elector of Saxony's need of gold. This prince, August the Strong, had ordered a certain Johann Böttger to obtain for him by the traditional methods of alchemy the required wealth to meet the demands of his own extravagances. Although Böttger's endeavours to raise the gold directly failed, he lighted upon the making of porcelain as another means of bringing in the princely income. Thus it was that the Albrecht Castle was in the year 1710 set at the disposal of the new enterprise by the Elector August.

The importance of this attainment of Böttger's in the history of the European potters can hardly be exaggerated. All Europe had been endeavouring in vain to produce ware as lovely as that which came from the Far East. Indeed, the best productions in Europe had got no further than what is known as "artificial porcelain," in the composition of which glass was an essential.

In the first place August the Strong had set up

experimental works in Dresden, his chief investigators being the alchemists Tschirnhaus and Böttger, and "it was to the glory of the latter to be the first to produce a porcelain like the Chinese, both as to the nature of the materials and in the appearance of its paste and glaze." Thirty years after the works were started in Meissen an art school was added to the amenities of the factory.

Amongst the artists who worked in painting the Meissen pottery, with its potters' mark of crossed swords, the names of two Hahnemann brothers appear in the records—that of Christian Gottfried who was appointed in 1741 *Maler Lehr-Bürsche*, painter apprentice, at the age of about twenty-one, and that of Christian August, whose appointment was a year later. The document referring to the second brother's appointment states that ". . . the Duke's Commissioner Hörold has appointed, with certain other painters, Christian August Hahnemann, born in Lauchstedt, twenty years of age; inasmuch as Commissioner Hörold has discovered in these persons a natural talent for painting, he hopes they will give useful service to the factory by working at the preparation of delicate flowers and landscapes." Hörold, the Court Commissioner, was at the time a man of considerable fame, during whose administration the reputation of the pottery reached its highest.

Our concern here is with Christian Gottfried, whose second marriage is recorded in the church register of Kotzschenbroda thus:

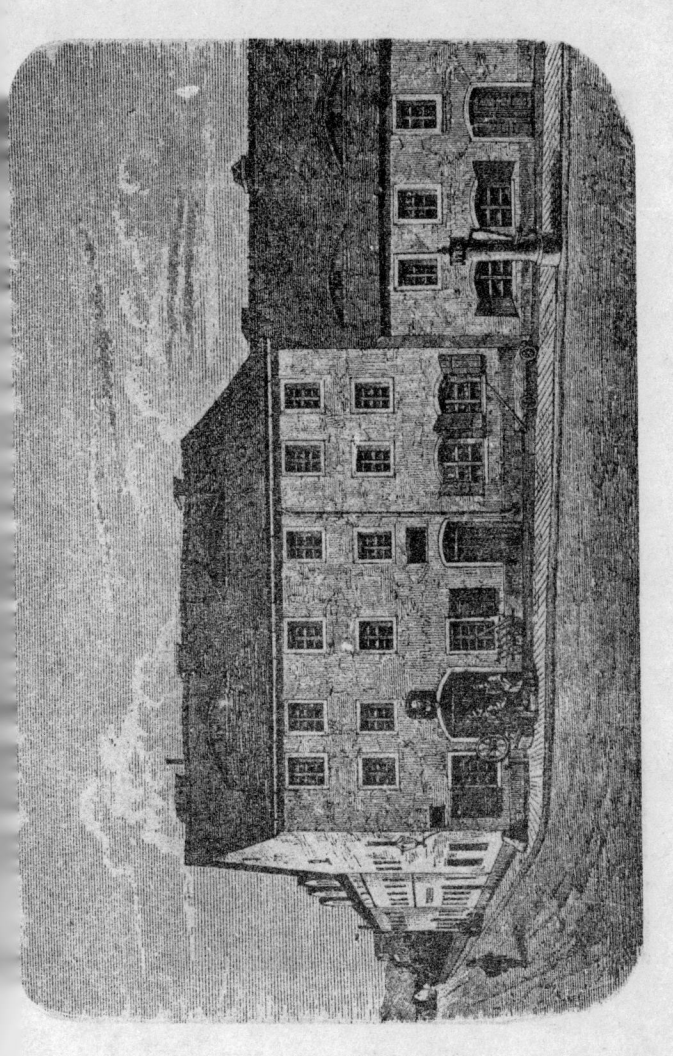

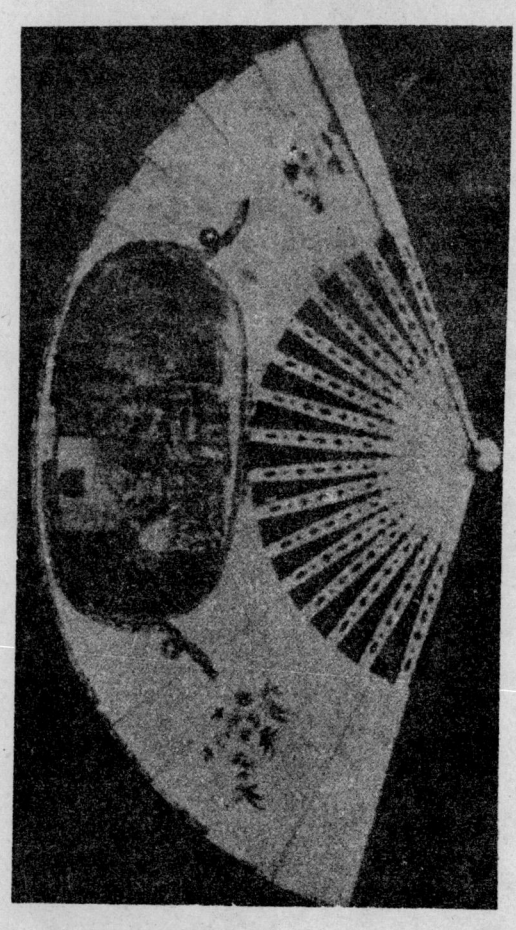

IVORY FAN PAINTED BY HAHNEMANN'S FATHER—HIS WEDDING GIFT TO HIS SON'S BRIDE

Faces page 17

THE MEISSEN PAINTERS

Christian Gottfried Hahnemann,
painter to His Majesty's porcelain factory
in Meissen, widower,
to Johanna Christiane,
only daughter of Johann Carl Spiessen,
Captain and Quartermaster, etc.

From this marriage sprang several children, the third being Christian Samuel. That Samuel Hahnemann's grandfather on his father's side, as well as his father and his uncle, Christian August, was also an artist, is indicated by several entries in the church register of Lauchstedt, in which his grandfather's name, Christoph Hahnemann, is recurrently followed by the epithet "the Painter." An autobiographical note by the son, tells us that Samuel Hahnemann's father, Christian Gottfried, published a small book on water-colour painting, whilst the many and varied illustrations to Christian Samuel Hahnemann's German biographer's exhaustive work include a photograph of an ivory fan painted by his father. It is clear, therefore, that the whole Hahnemann family was nurtured in the tradition of art work.

The house in which Samuel Hahnemann was born on 11th April, 1755, was a corner house of three stories, whitewashed, simple and compact, with wide windows admitting plenty of light. Perhaps it was largely on that account that his father purchased it. The actual building, known then as the Eck-haus, no longer stands, and a tall flaunting erection has taken its place. This, with its cut-away corner, in which stands a bust of Samuel Hahnemann, now serves as a restaurant to the neighbourhood. Over the entrance an inscription reads: "Here was born Christian Friedrich Samuel Hahnemann, the Founder of Homœopathy," followed by the date.

If it had not been for the Seven Years War, which commenced a year after the child's birth, the boyhood and youth of Samuel would have had to be written in quite a different vein. As it was, his early years bore the imprint of hardship. During that calamitous conflict a large consignment of the lovely Meissen ware was seized by King Frederick II of Prussia and was sold by him to a count who has been described as "an aristocratic profiteer," since he in his turn sold these works of art at a price increased by 40,000 thalers. The generals who took part were allowed to continue the havoc by further appropriations of the porcelain, whilst the Prussian king, with skilled labour drawn forcibly from Meissen, started a rival industry in Berlin. Yet, in spite of these bitter discouragements, the older centre survived, and through a varying standard of achievement, maintained that reputation for good workmanship which made the possession of its produce so enviable to these military robbers.

Needless to say, those who were engaged in the porcelain factory, whether as artists or as artisans, suffered acutely in consequence of this invasion. Thus it was that Samuel Hahnemann, the young son of the painter, endowed as he was with a thirst for knowledge, had to strive so ceaselessly to obtain for himself a sufficient opportunity for the acquirement of the rudiments of a good education. We are referring here to those studies which follow the elements of reading and writing, which arts were taught to the child by his father and mother together "whilst playing."

Nor was it in his childhood alone that Christian Samuel Hahnemann felt the impact of war upon his mind and spirit. In later years came the French occupation of Germany, and when a comparatively old man we hear him declaim against war as "the grave of science."

In the Franciscaneum, the town or Latin school of Meissen of those days, Hahnemann's admission appears in the register: "Christian Friedrich Samuel Hahnemann, son of the porcelain painter, 12 years old, Class 2, July 20, 1767." From a later testimony to the child's exceptional ability at this age we must either conclude that his father had educated him with great thoroughness or that the above records a readmission. For frequently in the opening phases of the boy's desire to learn his father took him from the town school, where, happily for the young student, his aptitude for foreign languages was early assisted. This withdrawal from study was insisted upon in order that the child's interests might be diverted from book learning to some field of occupation which, in after years, would yield him remuneration more readily than letters, or the professions to which letters lead. Even in the home study was discouraged. We read of the youthful student making a candlestick of clay in which to put his taper in some place of hiding, there to pore over his beloved books without being suspected, as he assuredly would have been had a candlestick been missed from its accustomed place on the shelf! On one occasion Samuel was sent to work in a grocery store at Leipzig, there to lay the foundation of experience needful for becoming a merchant. This occupation he left before long. Without permission he returned home fearfully to his parents. That his fears were justified is shown in that they were shared on his behalf by his mother, Johanna, who hid the boy in the house for several days till she had obtained the assurance of at least a moderately sympathetic reception from her husband. Little did the parents or the truant boy himself then dream that he would one day "defend his own dissertation from the Upper Chair," and become qualified to lecture on medicine in the city he had left.

Yet in later years this son had nothing critical to say of Gottfried Hahnemann, recognising that his father had good reason for his reluctance to encourage a studious spirit. "He had several other children to educate from his scanty income. That was sufficient excuse for the best of fathers." He says also that certain maxims of his father's not only remained keenly in his mind throughout his lifetime, but were remembered as having constituted the beginnings of some of his own most valued capacities. One of these: "Never be a passive listener or learner," Samuel Hahnemann tells us, followed him into the medical schools.

In some notes relating to members of the

THE MEISSEN PAINTERS

porcelain factory group, Professor Flügel mentions that the painter, before going to work, frequently put his son in a room with closed shutters, giving him a difficult sentence to think over, of which some account had to be given later. Apparently, in the professor's view, this practice of Gottfried Hahnemann's (though one we should hardly encourage other parents to imitate) contributed substantially to the son's ability to think with originality. The same disposition was borne out also by an old man in Meissen, who, years after, on hearing of the fame of the doctor, observed smilingly that, many a time when taking a walk with his father, Gottfried Hahnemann had remarked at a certain hour "I must go home now; I have a lesson to give to my son Samuel—a lesson in thinking." Yet, as Dr. Preuss, the Latin master in the Prince's School in Meissen, observes, even if the father was a stern disciplinarian, how much more influential must the intensely interesting work of Gottfried Hahnemann have been on the growing mind than any of the exercises imposed. Through the pen of Principal Albrecht we see Samuel as a boy wearing a queue, short trousers and shoes with buckles.

Fortunately for the youthful scholar, his teachers, during those intervals of schooling which he enjoyed, detected his exceptional powers. It was they who subsequently overcame, by practical measures, his father's unwillingness for him to continue his schooling—an unwillingness due beyond doubt to his poverty, for we cannot but believe that Gottfried Hahnemann, assured in his position and distinguished in his attainments, would otherwise have welcomed every opportunity for the development of the gifts latent in his children. This was done by offering the boy free tuition, and it was not long before they allowed the painter's son to balance that privilege by becoming what, in modern phraseology, would be called a pupil teacher. When only twelve years of age, Samuel was allowed by Magister Müller to assist the younger scholars with their first endeavours in Greek. Yet even this penetrating master may not have realised that the boy's early aptitude for languages foreshadowed a subsequent mastery of French, English, Italian, Greek, Hebrew, Arabic, and Spanish in addition to a peculiar force and fluency in his native German.

Happily for Samuel Hahnemann, in about 1770 this master, to whom he already owed so much, was transferred from the town school to the Prince's School in Meissen. This small township, renowned as a centre of science and art, was able to boast not a little of the educational facilities it offered. The Prince's School had been founded by the Elector Moritz of Saxony about 1545 with two others, to succeed the dispersed monastery of the Augustines, who had already had a school. It was now established as a "humanist" or classical gymnasium to board and train in the evangelical faith Saxon children of poor and rich alike. This democratic intention was stressed and scholarships founded, and its character remains unchanged to-day.

By what stages Gottfried Hahnemann was

persuaded finally to resign himself to sanction the development of his third child's capacities for learning, along lines which promised no short path to a remunerative occupation, is not known. There is no reason to exclude the possibility of a voluntary consent to such a step on the part of the father himself, in agreement with his wife. We cannot forget that this is the same man who shared with her the teaching of the children to read. Perhaps it was a pleasing recollection of these first lessons of his own infancy that led Samuel Hahnemann, when he himself had become a father, to take similar pleasure in making the studies of the arts of reading and writing of his own offspring "incredibly easy." He commenced teaching them with the aid of pictures, and held that "writing should be preceded by drawing," a method true to the history of the evolution of calligraphy.

Here we may close our sketch of the childhood and early years of Christian Samuel. Whilst we cannot altogether agree with Dr. Haehl that his was a "joyless youth," we cannot fail to recognise that its continuous conflict demanded a high courage and involved the suffering of countless pangs of apprehension, lest defeat should await his deeply cherished ambitions in the realm of study. These difficulties, including the necessity of being at times at variance with his father—no easy matter for a boy of tender years and sensitive mind—must sometimes have been almost insufferable. That his own future lifework was only dimly apprehended by the boy is probable; that he should be rendered fitted

for it, of whatever nature it might prove itself
to be, was his supreme resolution from a quite
abnormally early age. Yet however many obstacles there were to be overcome, surely there
must have been a peculiar compensation in the
fact that Magister Müller "loved him as if he
were his own child," and that, in spite of the
obvious preference sometimes accorded to him
by this master, his fellow scholars held him also
in their affection. In the brief autobiography,
from which we gain these glimpses of Samuel
Hahnemann in those early school days, we get a
delightful picture of the boy's master listening
in kindly fashion to his critical expositions of the
old writers during the private lessons given to
his boarders by Hahnemann.

If, moreover, the boy is in any true sense "the
father of the man," it is easy to believe that the
youthful Samuel Hahnemann was not altogether
lacking in happiness—he who in after years wrote
of the movements of the spider as "a kind of
flight, horizontally to and fro, and perpendicularly upwards," and added comments on entomology as a branch of natural history in which
the might, wisdom and goodness of God is to be
perceived. Similarly, Hahnemann wrote in those
later years of the supply of "the infinitesimal
needs of the little animals in the dust, invisible
to the sharpest human eye. . . ." Was he not
perhaps betraying in these expressions an early
acquired faculty for a sensitive observation and
awareness of those "inferior things and feeble
creatures," of which Ruskin speaks in his introduction to *German Popular Tales* as being

revealed to a child's "curiosity and companionship"?

If our conjecture is right, we may imagine that over and above the natural happiness which his home, with its artistic characteristics, yielded, in spite of some austerities and its restricted income, his excursions into the beautiful neighbourhood surrounding Meissen were touched with those delightful emotions belonging to the naturalist latent in each one of us, and which are bound up with those fresh and fairylike impressions peculiar to the closely-seen population and plant life of hedge and ditch. We know that as a boy he formed a herbarium. Indeed, around Meissen, with its vineyards and fertile tracts, lay one of the fairest of hilly landscapes.

CHAPTER II

STUDENTSHIP AND QUALIFICATION
Leipzig, Vienna, Hermannstadt, Erlangen, 1770-1779.

IN the year that Magister Müller was appointed to the Prince's School a petition was sent to the Prince Elector of Saxony by Gottfried Hahnemann, asking that his son might frequent the public lessons as "extraneus," or day scholar, and also "be entrusted to the instruction and special supervision of the third teacher of the same, M. Johann August Müller. . . ." The reply of the prince was favourable, and was expressed in the following terms to the rector of the "Landschool" in question:

> *"In consideration of the enclosed submissive petition of Christian Gottfried Hahnemann, we would graciously authorise that his son Christian Friedrich Samuel Hahnemann, as extraneus in our Landschool at Meissen, may come under the special supervision of the Collega Tertius, M. Johann August Müller, and may be present at the Lectiones Publicæ. We desire herewith that you take obedient notice, and make the necessary arrangements for it. That is Our Order."*

We can imagine with what stirrings of aspiration the boy's eyes scanned these sentences, for even in early years "hope deferred maketh the heart sick," and a desired end, when it is attained, becomes a veritable "tree of life." At least for a few years to come there was now the prospect of uninterrupted work for the eager student of sixteen years.

Before him there had passed through this school the poet and writer of fables, Gellert. Of Hahnemann's continued interest in Gellert's writings over a number of years we have evidence in his choice of a verse of his with which to introduce one of his own larger works. Lessing, too, had been amongst the scholars of the Prince's School.

When Hahnemann entered the school there was much competition for admission. For this being open to the children of parents in every profession and trade, many had to start as day scholars and become scholarship-boarders later. Such was the case with Hahnemann, who later became "famulus" to Müller. The discipline was "conventual," that is to say, the school inherited from its monastic predecessor a marked strictness, expulsions being effected for what might be regarded in these days as "minor offences."

The boys in the prosperous days of the school were provided with a uniform including a scholar's "shoulder" gown, and we find in the old records that "38 ells of cloth were provided for each four scholars" for the purpose. Over the entrance to the school were inscribed the words: "To Christ and Learning." The motto, taken from the writings of Horace, "Sapere Aude," "Dare to be wise," is now to be found in three places; one of these, on an old playground wall, was certainly read and remembered by Samuel Hahnemann. We find these words on the title page of one of his most important works.

There was one important direction in which the circumstances of his home life at this period most probably influenced the young Hahnemann's career. In the records of the porcelain factory his uncle, Christian August, is described as an "Indianischer Blumenmaler" ("flower-painter") and a painter of "delicate flowers and landscapes," and this description almost certainly applies to his father also. Hahnemann himself has told us that botany, with mathematics and geometry, were the only regular school subjects in which he took special interest—and this in spite of his genius for languages.

If we examine the beautiful collection of Meissen porcelain on view at the Victoria and Albert Museum in London, we may observe that the Chinese flowers (which came by way of the East Indies) still in vogue in 1742, when the brothers Hahnemann began their career as painters in Meissen, were soon after that date superseded by "German" or native European flowers. These were, especially in the earlier period, largely copied from prints and of a composite and conventional type, but they were also in many cases copies from nature. Favourites are rose, peony, tulip, lily, pansy, cornflower, fritillary, convolvulus. (It was a rule of the factory, alas, that artists must not put their names on the objects adorned with their designs.)

It would be natural that Samuel Hahnemann's father and uncle would wish to have, besides garden flowers, some of the wild species of the locality for use and enjoyment in connection with their art. It may therefore well have been the case that it was through these circumstances that the young Samuel acquired his love of botany, and as a further result his interest in the medical properties of the various plants and herbs. In the eighteenth century there were many German herbalists, and the medical lore of flowers and herbs was especially honoured in Saxony. We may even guess that the boy in some of his rambles, perhaps while gathering a nosegay for the two artists, may have had occasionally one of these wise collectors for his companion, and have fed his boyish mind on his stores of traditional wisdom.

During the early growing years of Christian Samuel Hahnemann we have already noted the stern struggle for its own existence that the scholarly side of his disposition had to experience. Regarding the later years of his studies we have a fragment revealing the strenuous nature of his student life. It appears in a letter to a philological student who had consulted him regarding mental overstrain. Hahnemann in reply wrote: "Mental exertion and study are unnatural occupations for young people whose bodily development is not yet complete, especially for those who are endowed with sensitive feelings. This nearly cost me my life during the period from fifteen to twenty years of age." The observation follows: "Strenuous study and pro-

MEDICAL QUALIFICATION

found thought absorb a greater portion of life's energy than is required to thresh corn in a barn."

In 1775 Samuel Hahnemann was preparing to leave the Prince's School. He chose as the subject of his farewell dissertation "The Wonderful Construction of the Human Hand." Until recently no copy of this oration could be traced, but thanks to Dr. Preuss of the Prince's School, Meissen, it has now been found and printed with a German translation opposite to its original Latin and a scholarly preface by the same pen. It is our privilege to quote from it in English for the first time.

"The *Entlassungstag* was the great day of farewell speeches," writes Stephen Hobhouse (to whom we owe the English translation), "when in the festal Assembly Hall—the *Aula*—there would be gathered together scholars and staff past and present, admiring parents and illustrious patrons and other friends, to listen to the oratorical exploits of the fortunate boys, who were singled out for this distinction as a solemn winding up of their school career. The speakers were supposed to stand forth in the dignity of the scholar's gown of good black cloth, which was then the regulation costume; though it is likely that in the general poverty and desolation which had at that time overspread Saxony, owing to the wars of Frederick the Great, the provision of the gown had largely fallen into abeyance, and that the boys may have had to appear in the most suitable clothing that their parents could provide.

"On this particular occasion one of the most prominent among these young speakers was Christian Friedrich Samuel Hahnemann. He may indeed have been actually the head boy, 'Primus Omnium,' to whom alone in modern practice the duty of a Latin Oration has been assigned. As he had assisted in the teaching under Rector Müller, it is probable that he was equipped with the distinction of the scholar's shoulder gown, even though its use may have now become rare.

"Samuel had just passed his twentieth birthday and was the pride of his parents as well as of his school for his remarkable gifts, especially in the domain of foreign languages.

"We will now leave the young Hahnemann to speak for himself, constructing in our mind's eye a picture of him standing out prominently upon the school *bema* or platform, with his teachers behind him and an appreciative audience on the seats in front, their eyes fixed on his thin delicate figure, with its striking head and with a demeanour expressive at once of a vigorous self-confidence and a modesty befitting the solemnity of the occasion."

Marked with both the warmth of enthusiasm at its opening and the keenness of clear thinking as it proceeds, the *Oratio* commences with the words:

"None of you, most honourable and learned auditors, can doubt that the existence of God may be known and understood from the

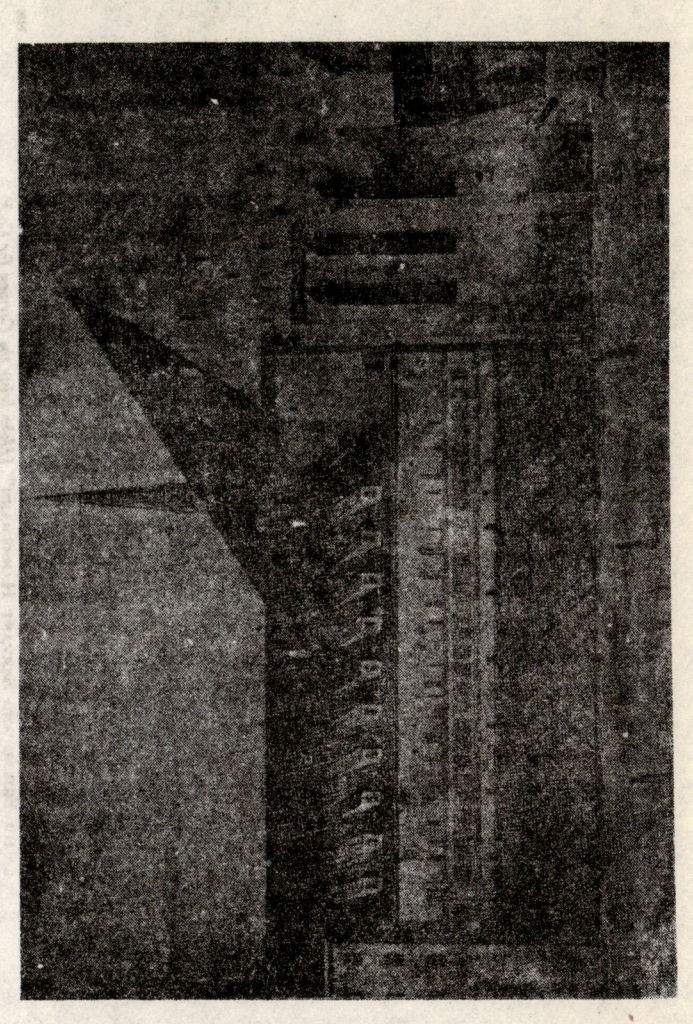

Das ● Probirt man in der Glüth,
Den Lob die Klinge gut,
Die Krafft der ● durch Gifft,
Das ● wenn es der Sturm Wind trifft.
Soldaten ●● in der Schlacht
Der Jungfern Keuschheit ● der Nacht
Bei Freunden ist der Probe
Wenn wir in höchsten nöthen son ─

Meißen d. 9ten Octobr
1782.

Dem Herrn Crafter zum Andendem
schrieb diß gutter kan
sein Freund und Diener
─ Hanemann ─

THE DEDICATION BELOW THE 'REBUS' READS: "FOR THE [BOOK'S] OWNER THIS KEEPSAKE WROTE, AS HE BEST HE CAN,
HIS FRIEND AND SERVANT HAHNEMANN" (*Hahn* being the German for *Cock*)[1]

mechanism of His universe; and yet I think I may to-day assert that it is above all else in the construction of the human body that the wonderful wisdom and beneficence of the Supreme Being is most radiantly shown forth. For in each and every limb He has shown such an almost incredible skill in craftsmanship and such an exquisite art that anyone who dares to cast blame on the least thing in the composition of our bodies may rightly and deservedly be considered not only a fool but deprived of all sense and insight. Moreover, as a man is easily the chief of all living creatures, so the dignity and perfection of his body is far above that of theirs."

The passage following enters into a consideration of the adaptation of their bodily form to the nature and the needs of different animals, especially as regards self-defence, in which the hands excel. The essay then continues:

"What shall I say of the arts discovered with the help of the hands or of the clothing made by them? What of the buildings constructed either for human comfort or for protection or for necessity? Moreover, what laws would we possess, what products of genius, if we were without hands? The hands are indeed the benefactors that enable us to hold converse with Plato and with Aristotle, with Hippocrates and with Galen, and with others who were prominent in the ancient world. . ."

Comment is then made on the ability of the hand to play the part of various tools, also to the thinness of the flesh which "the Divine Artist" has placed between the fingers on the inner side, so that they can be closed for swimming and for drinking.

"Could one believe," he asks, "that the famous Diogenes of Sinope would have thrown away his cup unless he had been able to drink water from a hand thus compressed?" From here the *Oratio* goes forward in a more precisely anatomical strain.

The speech closes with the words:

> "Let me, honoured and learned auditors, at length conclude by saying that I hold myself to have proved to you, as far as the weakness of my poor capacities has permitted me, that the mechanism of our hands has been elaborated and brought to perfection by the All-wise Creator of the world with a marvellous and divine craftsmanship. And you, finally, my good comrades in the school, let me admonish and beseech, to venerate with me that Supreme Providence which has assuredly given a clear revelation of itself as much in the least of created beings as in the wisest and mightiest of the angels. For believe me, He has equipped and adorned our minds with understanding and intelligence for no other reason, save that we may gain a knowledge of Himself—a knowledge which we may have by contemplating ourselves and other things that He has created; and this wonderful sight is not possible to any other species of creatures."

The young Saxon student, it will be realised, was speaking before the theory of evolution had been propounded. The foundation of the idealist view of creation, as revealing a divine *purpose* in all its works, was no doubt derived by Hahnemann partly from the example and teaching of Christian Gottfried, his father, and also from the greatest of the pre-Christian philosophers, Plato and Aristotle, whom he names. These Stephen Hobhouse refers to as his models of wisdom, "for" he continues, "their outlook, or 'Weltanschauung,' is through and through what is known as 'teleological,' that is, everything in nature is explained as providentially adapted to some special end or purpose." This view we are reminded was also taken by Galen, though Galen uses the term "Nature" instead of God almost uniformly.

"It is interesting," the same writer adds, "to recall that two of the greatest nineteenth century British anatomists and surgeons, Sir Charles Bell of Edinburgh and Sir George Humphry of Cambridge, also wrote works of considerable literary charm upon the Human Hand, dealing with the hand's wonderful adaptability for its manifold functions. Bell's book has as its title *The Hand, its mechanism and vital endowments, as evincing* [providential] *design*, which almost exactly describes Hahnemann's earlier essay."

"As a literary work," Stephen Hobhouse continues, "this is a most striking performance for a young man, and Hahnemann has caught very aptly the special idiom and characteristics of Cicero, chief among Latin rhetorical and philosophical authors. The writer's material I have discovered to have been taken to a very considerable extent from the first and last books of the *De Usu Partium* of Galen, the father of mediæval medicine. I am inclined to think that he used the original Greek for his material, instead of the much commoner Latin version of Galen; and this he has done very skilfully, for, with very few exceptions, there is no verbal dependence. Indeed, the high standard of scholarship then prevailing in the Prince's School makes it natural that he should consult the Greek text. It will be noticed by anyone reading the *Oratio* that Hahnemann states quite frankly that he took his subject-matter from the 'Physici' (*i.e.* the 'natural philosophers' or 'scientific writers'); and he boldly adopts the sentence of Galen, in which that writer says that it is only the hands which enable us to hold converse with Plato, Aristotle, Hippocrates, and others of the ancients, merely adding to these names that of Galen himself."

As was and is still the custom at the Prince's School, the Latin oration was followed by a valedictory Ode. This was intended to express the gratitude of the outgoing pupil to all who had helped him in his studies, not only in the School but also in his home. This Ode, though it was not usual to do so, Hahnemann wrote in French. In it is expressed a spirit of gratitude beyond the formal acknowledgement of indebtedness expected, and it contains also several autobiographical fragments. It commences with the words:

"Je viens Lui consacrer les feux de ma jeunesse
Chantant Ses immortels bienfaits."

"I come to consecrate to Him the fire of my youth
Hymning His eternal blessings."

"Into these abodes of peace, this devout Seminary
Thou dost lead my steps . . .
Where I have been gathering honey of the Fine Arts."

In further lines he calls his school years "the beautiful era" and the precincts of the School "those delicious courts." The feeling for this harmony, near at hand and afar, this "concinnatio" of all creation, went with him, as Dr. Preuss stresses, throughout his life.

Writing of the "Oratio" which he was kind enough to read, Dr. Poynton, the Public Orator of Oxford University, says: "The Latin is clear and has character. The construction is good. The whole piece has a directness and force which compensate for minor defects of phraseology. It is difficult to follow Tully [*i.e.* Cicero] in this field."

It is remarkable that even a senior pupil at a public school should have been a student of the old medical authorities. No one to-day, his translator into English reminds us, in school or university would read either Hippocrates or Galen. Ernst von Brunnow, whose opportunities for talk with Hahnemann in later years were numerous, throws a light on this unusual feature in his school career. "Besides an eagerness for the classical literature of the ancients," he writes, "the growing youth displayed an ardent inclination for the study of the natural sciences and of medicine. The necessary time for these studies was willingly allowed him by the benevolent principal, though this indulgence was contrary to the strict plan of the school." That the conception of the world, of men, and of God, held by these ancient Greek philosophers had not only a powerful but also a lasting influence on Samuel Hahnemann, is shown in his later life and writings.

In this choice of a subject, as he was preparing to go to a medical school, we have a hint of good things to come. With only as many thalers as years in his possession—this "twenty thalers" being the last contribution made by his father towards his qualification for what was to be his life's work—Hahnemann left Meissen in the spring of 1775 to enter the University in Leipzig. This town was then not only the centre of intellectual activity for the Duchy of Saxony, but also for the larger part of Germany, and, Haehl adds, "for the whole of cultured Europe."

Needless to say, his last allowance from home did not admit of any extravagance in his way of living, and indeed could not for very long meet even the supply of necessities. It was only by adding to the tasks of studentship the work of translating and teaching that the expenses of a medical education could finally be met. To a wealthy young Greek Hahnemann gave lessons in French and German, whilst the works he chose to render into his own language were at this time chiefly English. In his first year Hahnemann produced a Latin poem in praise of Professor Zeune, whose lectures "disclosed the treasures of Rome and Hellas." This was presented under the inscription, "From three of his audience."

Besides taking exercise, which the student had by now realised to be essential, if he was to preserve a measure of health sufficient for the work to which he had set his mind, Samuel Hahnemann had few if any recreations. He enjoyed, however, certain privileges. As at the Prince's School, by the wise provision of his master, he had only attended those classes which he felt would be of use to him, so here in the University Hahnemann expended none of his energies on lectures which seemed unlikely to yield him the knowledge he required. This exercise of his selective faculty was not for the purpose of economy, strictly necessary though economy must have been, since Bergrat Dr. Pörner, who had known him in Meissen, was usually able to obtain for him free access to the lectures. His one strong complaint against the Medical School was not directed against the Professors or their orations, but to the fact that it offered no field for clinical work. Leipzig at that time had no hospital.

In consequence of this deficiency it was not

long before Samuel Hahnemann was packing up his spare belongings in preparation for migrating to Vienna. This was in spite of the heavy expense incidental to such a move. With 68 gulden and 12 kreuzer in his pockets, he set out for a new and wider world of experience, this time to be found in Vienna.

In the Austrian capital there were already two hospitals. The oldest was that of the Brothers of Mercy, whose head physician, Dr. Quarin—also Physician-in-ordinary to the Empress Maria Theresa—had supplied the Emperor Joseph II with the plans for the second, the General Hospital. To this was attached a Maternity Hospital and a Foundling Home. Besides these there was also associated with the General Hospital an Asylum for the insane known as the Narrenturm or Lunatic Tower.

Although there was so far no hospital in Europe that surpassed the General Hospital in Vienna, both in its size and the excellence of its accommodation, the eager student elected to enter that of the Brothers of Mercy, and this in spite of his own Lutheran upbringing. Hahnemann had good reason for this step in the fact that Dr. Quarin was there in residence. This teacher, who was six times elected Rector of the Vienna University, now proved a second Johann Müller to Samuel Hahnemann, showing him a similar confidence and affection, as was abundantly evidenced. That there was no hope of remuneration for the exceptional opportunities for learning bestowed upon the promising undergraduate, Dr. Quarin could not have failed to realise.

This helps us to estimate better his valuation of Hahnemann's capacities. Writing of this time, Hahnemann says: "I am indebted for my medical instinct to the Hospital of the Brothers of Mercy of Leopoldstadt, or rather to the practical genius of Dr. von Quarin, physician-in-ordinary to the Prince's family. I had his friendship, I could almost say his love; I was the only one at that time whom he allowed to accompany him to his private patients."

It is not difficult to imagine the happiness with which Samuel Hahnemann, now almost twenty-two years of age, availed himself of these facilities for gaining insight and increasing his practical knowledge. This personal touch with actual practice must have been all the more appreciated after the dearth of anything but theoretic teaching in Leipzig. But there was now, unfortunately, no time for his previously pursued remunerative occupations. Whilst he could accept opportunities for learning, Hahnemann could not look to another for his personal support. As his financial reserves dwindled, it became necessary for him after only nine months in the favourable circumstances of Vienna to cast about in his mind for another step in his student career. It appears from the "autobiography" that the time spent in Vienna might have been longer, but for "a malicious trick" which had been played upon Hahnemann in Leipzig, robbing him of a sum of money earned in that city. Writing of this he says, "repentance demands reconciliation, and I will be silent about name and circumstances." The nature of the step decided upon was shaped for him by the friendly doctor to whom he already owed so much encouragement.

It happened at this time that the Governor of Transylvania had come to Vienna to receive instructions from the Imperial Government there, and it was to this man, Samuel von Brukenthal, like Hahnemann a Saxon and a Protestant, that Dr. Quarin introduced the student of medicine. As a result, an attractive post was offered to him, though one somewhat aside from his chosen line of study. In the Governor's home in Hermannstadt was a large library needing careful arrangement and, besides this, a collection of valuable coins requiring classification. These tasks were entrusted to the medical candidate. As an indication of the extent to which Dr Quarin must have commended his already acquired medical abilities, Samuel Hahnemann, though not yet possessing a degree, was engaged as medical adviser to the Governor and the officers of his household, and also allowed to practice in the township "as a young disciple of Æsculapius."

For a year and nine months he thus lived in Hermannstadt, a town which has been described as being at that time the frontier of German influence and West-European culture. Albrecht tells of an incident in the doctor's experience when travelling in Transylvania. He "encountered a lady of high rank in an hotel; the landlady in providing dinner for her guests neglected the fire, and in a short time the whole house was in a blaze. Everyone thought of his own safety, no one attending to the lady, whose apartments were in the upper story. Hahnemann rushed through the midst of the flames, returned with the rescued lady, and also saved her heavy trunk. Being satisfied of her safety, he immediately entered the stage and drove away." The same biographer also records a similar event in later life in Lobkowitz, near Dresden, when Hahnemann, although by then the father of four children, "encountered all risks" and was the means of extinguishing a dreadful fire which had broken out.

Whether Hahnemann travelled from Vienna to Hermannstadt with the Governor does not appear, but it is known that, three days after Brukenthal's arrival, Hahnemann was admitted to the Freemason's Lodge of "St. Andrew of the Three Leaves," of which the Governor was a member.

During this time spent in the house of his kindly patron, Hahnemann must have experienced a relaxation from financial anxiety and circumstances of comfort unknown to him till that period, so that we can regard his stay in Hermannstadt as partaking partly of the nature of a rest, in spite of the numerous and varied responsibilities he had undertaken. Of this time in Hermannstadt Hahnemann wrote:

> "I had the opportunity of learning several other necessary languages, and of acquiring knowledge of some collateral sciences in which I was still lacking. I arranged and catalogued the Governor's matchless collection of ancient

coins as well as his library, practised medicine for a year and nine months in this populous town, and then departed, although very unwillingly, from these honourable people. . ."

From this retreat Hahnemann withdrew in 1779 only to pursue more closely the requirements of his vocation, the time having arrived for the practising student to become the qualified physician. This qualification he sought in Erlangen.

The thesis by which, after passing the prescribed *Examen rigorosum*, Hahnemann's degree was obtained, was entitled: "A Summary of the conditions of Cramp according to cause and cure." It was submitted "by consent of the Friedrich Alexander University, under the Rectorate of His Serene Highness the Prince and Sovereign Karl Alexander, Margrave of Brandenburg, Duke of Prussia and Silesia, for the rightful purpose of gaining the degree of Doctor in the Medical Faculty, by a public examination by an Academic Board." As was customary, the essay, which was in Latin, was first handed in in writing and afterwards "defended verbally." The degree was conferred at Erlanger in August, 1779.

The difference in the standards of medical training and accomplishment in Hahnemann's day and our own is indicated in the fact that the Medical School in Leipzig, the most famous University in Germany, had offered him little or nothing but lectures and book learning, without even the promise of clinical experiencè elsewhere, and also in that Brukenthal, a high official of the state in Austria, had allowed Samuel Hahnemann, before he had taken his full qualification, to practise both in his household and in the territory over which he was Governor.

Haehl, commenting on the self-imposed character of Hahnemann's close application to chemistry, throws a further light on the state of things in this connection. "Chemistry," he writes, "was [in those days] left to the apothecaries, and microscopy to the specialists in natural science." In fact, the course of medical training prescribed at the University did not at that time include these subjects: even so famous a University as the one at Heidelberg did not introduce microscopy and chemistry in the syllabus of their medical students until 1845.

CHAPTER III

FIRST PRACTICE AND MARRIAGE

Hettstedt, Dessau, Gommern, Dresden, Leipzig,
1779-1789.

AT Hettstedt, among the Harz Mountains, Samuel Hahnemann at twenty-four years commenced his first practice as a qualified doctor. This little place, in the Saxon County of Mansfeld, with its three or four thousand inhabitants, was the scene of the copper mining industry, and offered Hahnemann opportunities for studying metallurgy. From the 12th century copper had been found here. Hahnemann's first original essays produced at the time appear in Krebs' *Medical Observations* recording his experience in a particular type of fever observed over a period of nine months in Quenstädt in the Mansfeld district. The opinions expressed in them already betray that directness of conviction and indifference to the consequences of an utter sincerity which were to characterise the author throughout his life:

"I am not daring too much," he states, "when I maintain that epidemics, in the beginning, are largely illnesses of isolated individuals which could easily be subjugated ; and that they only degenerate into an angel of destruction by carelessness and ignorance. . . . If I omit a prolonged spell of unhealthy weather conditions, penury and poverty, the remaining fault falls almost entirely on institutions, nurses and doctors, who alone by their combined bad behaviour are able to change moderate epidemics into serious ones."

"From the time of Hippocrates to our own day," Singer in his *Short History of Medicine* remarks, "the subject of Epidemics has occupied the attention of physicians." The *Hippocratic Collection* contains a treatise on epidemics, and certainly Hahnemann must be regarded as a notable figure in this line of succession. Already in 1782 he is declaiming against the unhygienic conditions under which the people are compelled to live; and later years produced, as we shall find, several works on the question, in which he anticipated many modern preventive methods.

The fact of Hettstedt being in his native state of Saxony appears to have been the chief attraction to Hahnemann. Regarding this step he wrote: "The instinctive longing of a Swiss for his rugged Alps cannot be more irresistible than that of a Saxon for his native land." But the small opportunities offered him there, both as regards his work and intellectual intercourse, soon led Hahnemann to seek a sphere of usefulness elsewhere. At the end of nine months, in the spring of 1781, a new home was made in Dessau, not more than fifty kilometres distant from Hettstedt, a move with important consequences.

FIRST PRACTICE AND MARRIAGE

Dessau, the largest town as well as the capital of what has been since 1918 the Free State of Anhalt, remains, in spite of its industrial character, a quiet and attractive place in flat though prettily wooded country on the banks of the rapid Mulde, one of the chief tributaries of the Elbe, whose mighty stream it joins some two miles lower down. Apart from some of its numerous and handsome public buildings, nearly all the houses appear to have been rebuilt since Hahnemann's day. It still, however, with its palaces, picture galleries and gardens, bears the impress of the paternal autocrats who took a pride in making their beautiful possessions accessible to the subjects over whom they ruled.

Here Hahnemann was to meet a young woman several years his junior, who proved herself to be from the first one of character and charm. This was Johanna Leopoldine Henriette Küchler, step-daughter of Herr Häseler. an apothecary, himself the son of an architect. With him the young physician during his "hours of leisure," as he characteristically put it in after years, worked experimentally in chemistry. In 1781, to Henriette Küchler, at the age of seventeen, Hahnemann became betrothed. There may be seen in Dessau some delightful silhouettes of the dignified figure of the Dessau *Apotheker*, Herr Häseler, and his family. Jn. Gothard Küchler, Henriette's father, whose widow Herr Häseler had married, had preceded Häseler at the *Mohren-Apotheke*.

The *Mohren-Apotheke* or Moor-Pharmacy, which belonged to Herr Häseler and afterwards to his widow and grandson, still exists to-day in modern buildings, apparently in the same busy street as it used to be. Though the fact of Hahnemann's connection with it is hardly known even to the present proprietor, the original painted-wood figure of the dusky old Moor, with his bow and arrows, his turban and his red and green feather-petticoat, still stands over the shop door, and homœopathic remedies are a principal feature of the stock.

If the views of the principal Dessau antiquarian are correct, the sign of the Moor, which is said to be a favourite one for a pharmacy in the principality of Anhalt, owes its origin to the fact that in the sixteenth and seventeenth centuries (as can be seen from many well-known portrait groups) kings and princes had a liking for young Moors or Negroes as pages, and this was especially the case in the family of Nassau-Orange (that of our William III) with whom the rulers of Anhalt had married. The *Mohren-Apotheke* in Dessau, founded in 1695, supplied the needs of the Anhalt Court.

As a rule the German pharmacies are picturesquely called after various animals. Thus in Dessau the earliest establishment licensed (about 1600) was the *Löwe*—Lion, then came the *Adler*—Eagle, the *Mohr*, and the *Einhorn*—Unicorn. To these have been added in recent years the *Paulus*, *Bär*—Bear, and *Hirsch*—Stag, and this number is held to suffice for Dessau with its population of well over 50,000.

The Apotheker, owing to his training and his privileged position, was an important person.

FIRST PRACTICE AND MARRIAGE

Readers of Goethe's epic of domestic life, *Hermann and Dorothea*, will remember that the Clergyman, the Innkeeper and the Chemist, the *Herr Pfarrer*, the *Herr Wirt* and the *Herr Apotheker*, appear as the three principal personages of the little South German town where the scene is laid, and that the Apotheker discourses on the expense of giving a new coat of gold paint to the Archangel Michael, who presided over the entrance to his shop.

The Government in many of the German States fixed prices and regulated the supply of dangerous drugs; while a Standing Committee of Physicians examined in Latin and in pharmaceutical chemistry the candidates for the position of Apotheker, who had previously served for a term of years as apprentices and assistants (*Gesellen*). In spite of all this training there were many complaints, at any rate until comparatively modern times, of insufficiency of knowledge on the part of Apothekers.

At about this time we know that Hahnemann visited his home, for we have a delightful "rebus" from his pen dated Meissen, 9th October, 1782. The lines, with their picture-words, conceived in a light vein embody serious thoughts. In translation they read thus:

"For *gold* the test by fire is made:
True rings the steel of perfect *blade:*
From poisons *healing draughts* are riven:
Ships prove their worth when tempest driven:
The soldier's *heart* 's revealed in fight:
The maiden's chastity *by* night:

While friendship's test will ever *be*
The touch*stone* of adversity.

We have put in italics the words shown in picture form, the colours of which are still vivid and harmonious—the disc and sword of the first two lines in gold, the medicine-bottle white with brown liquid and a red stopper, the hearts rose-pink, the ship and the stone brown, whilst the eggs (forming the interior of two words) are white.

On the 17th November in the same year, two years after their engagement, Samuel Hahnemann and Henriette Küchler were married at the Church of St. John in Dessau, the doctor of twenty-eight to the apothecary's daughter of nineteen.

The first home to which the newly married pair went was in the neighbouring township of Gommern, where Samuel Hahnemann had, since his coming to Dessau, been appointed as Medical Officer of Health. He was, therefore, near enough to continue the experiments which he had undertaken at his father-in-law's house.

Two years after their marriage Samuel Hahnemann's father, Christian Gottfried, died. In a slender autobiography, penned some time after, the doctor wrote of him:

" 'To act and live without show or pretence' was his most notable precept. He was frequently present, attentive and unobserved, when something good was to be accomplished. In his actions he discriminated with the utmost nicety between the noble and the base and with a correctness that showed how truly admirable was the practical delicacy of his feelings. In this he was my teacher. His ideas on the foundation laws of the universe, on the dignity of mankind, and its lofty destiny, seemed consistent in every way with his habits of living. This gave me the direction of my inner life."

"Here," writes Stephen Hobhouse, in his sketch of Gottfried Hahnemann, "we have a glimpse of a good and a gifted man, whose character evidently did much to mould that of his great son. It has been hitherto a real loss, that we knew no more about him. And now at last the deficiency is partially supplied, through a search made through the archives of the famous Meissen factory of 'Dresden China.' This search was set in motion by the writer, when on a visit to the beautiful Saxon town in October, 1931. . . . In the factory records we find that Christian Gottfried Hahnemann died in 1784, and during the last two and a half years of his life he wrote a series of some six letters, addressed to the Saxon Elector through the Director, Count Marcolini, of which copies have now come to light. The circumstances which produced them were as follows.

"The Sultan of Turkey had ordered from the factory a large porcelain table. It was found impossible, as in other cases of attempts to produce very large porcelain articles, to bring it out of the oven without cracks appearing in the finished work. The large recumbent goat of eighteenth century Meissen porcelain, now in the Victoria and Albert Museum, South Kensington, provides an example of this defect.

"Hahnemann, though primarily a painter, thought he could find the means of remedying this misfortune, and was encouraged to do so by the Prince and by the Director. The letters discovered refer to his efforts in this field. They exhibit him as tirelessly making one experiment after another, confident that he will succeed in the end, in spite of several failures and the opposition of the chemists of the factory. His second son, Samuel August, who had had an apothecary's training, gave him assistance."

The letter which Christian Gottfried wrote before his retirement reads:

"At the Prince Elector's Saxon Porcelain Factory in Meissen, November and December, 1784.

"To the Lord High Chamberlain, His Excellency Count Marcolini, acting Privy Councillor and Director of the Meissen Porcelain Factory.

"Already in the month of August of the present year, have I humbly laid before your Excellency a complete outline of my invention of a method of giving a firmer consistency to the material of the porcelain; and I have begged your Excellency most graciously to dispense with my further services, because of the serious failing of my eyesight.

"Although the allowance [of money] graciously made to me by your Excellency's orders was withdrawn and I was transferred to painting again, nevertheless, most arduous as the work is for me under present circumstances, I have not in any respect lost sight of the high interests of the gracious ruler of my country. On the contrary, I have ceaselessly striven to discover by what means the expense caused by this invention of mine can be turned in the future to the best advantage; and how it may be practicable by the best available methods to clear away completely the hindrances, which it has hitherto appeared impossible to remove. . . .

"I will accordingly leave it to your Excellency's honourable judgment to hand over the execution of this experiment to the person, whose high privilege it is to possess your Excellency's confidence. I am far from putting myself forward as the only man to undertake this task. Still, I am perfectly convinced that by this method, provided my suggestions are followed, a much more successful experiment than the ones already made is bound to result.

"Only—all the renewed expenditure of effort remains notwithstanding quite fruitless, because all the factory chemists ['*Arcanists*'] do their best to oppose and prevent the experiment merely because the discovery is not their own. But, whether on that account the credit of the factory and the high interests of our most gracious Elector should be neglected, will be a matter for your Excellency to decide.

"I remain, as long as I live, your Excellency's

humble and obedient servant, [signed] Christian Gottfried Hahnemann."

This letter is immediately followed in the archives of the Factory by the statement, "On the 15th of this month the painter, Christian Gottfried Hahnemann, died in the sixty-sixth year of his age, after having been ill for only a week."

"I think it will be agreed," the writer we are quoting goes on to say, "that the newly discovered matter just summarised and the painter's last letter which I have translated, give us an insight into the character of a remarkable man, . . . one who could leave his more congenial tasks to try and remedy apparently unsurmountable defects in a kindred sphere of art production, and who could persist to the last, in spite of serious ailment and the sacrifice of his private income, in the face of the jealousy and opposition of his fellow-craftsmen . . . and, finally, an artist of sufficient humility and selflessness to hand on to others, when he felt his strength failing and his life ebbing away, what he believed to be the secret of his ultimate success, urging that he was not himself indispensable to attain the desired goal.

"May we not say that most of the characteristics exemplified in these records of Christian Gottfried Hahnemann are to be found also in the great physician and pioneer, who was his son? And we may well credit the son, when he tells us, that it was his father's example

FIRST PRACTICE AND MARRIAGE

and precepts which gave him the direction of his inner life."

It was in Gommern that Samuel Hahnemann commenced his translation of two volumes by the French chemist Demachy. This contribution to science marked the commencement of his own career as a chemist, in which sphere he was to win distinguished recognition. Demachy himself had already been made a member of the Berlin Academy, as well as of his own French Academy in Paris. This book was likely to meet with a keen reception beyond the borders of his own country, as it concerned matters of universal importance to trade. Its design was so to encourage the chemical industry as to break down the monopolies of those firms which, especially in Holland, guarded their secrets with assiduity. It concerned in fact "the wholesale manufacture of chemicals, or the science of preparing chemicals in factories."

In addition to the task of a translator, Hahnemann took upon himself the responsibility of annotating the original work. Besides footnotes he added supplements giving independent references. A review in the then leading Journal of Chemistry in Germany, Crell's *Annals*, reads as follows:

"If ever a work was worth translating, it is certainly the present one, which, fortunately for all its readers, fell into the hands of one who has made it more complete." This translation was published in 1785, by which time we find Hahnemann and his wife in Dresden.

Gommern had offered him no facilities for earning save by practising medicine, of the true application of which he was increasingly convinced he was not yet aware. No less informed than his colleagues, indeed in some respects as regards the auxiliary sciences better equipped than many, he was dismayed at the state of ignorance with which the medical profession appeared to be content. It had become imperative therefore that other sources of livelihood should be found; and hence his migration, with his wife and daughter Henrietta, to Dresden. The tenderness of his relationship to the first inhabitant of the family cot is hinted at in a little lullaby which Hahnemann composed:

> "Sleep daughter soon!
> The bunting pipes in the wood·
> Gaily it hops on the snow
> And quietly sleeps on the bare twigs,
> Sleep soon!"

In the capital, frequented as it was by notable persons, Dresden being the centre of courtly festivities and military gatherings, Hahnemann, bent upon deeper issues, remained for four years. These years, he observes, passed with remarkable swiftness. Amongst Hahnemann's friendships there formed was that with the philologist, John Aristophanes Adelung. This man held the post of Superintendent of the Electoral Library, and was the compiler of a work in five volumes, a history of the languages and dialects of the world. The use of the library was of

FIRST PRACTICE AND MARRIAGE

great importance to Hahnemann. It was here that he met the famous French chemist Lavoisier, who was mainly responsible for the conversion of scientific men to the doctrine that "matter can neither be created nor destroyed by chemical agencies," or, as we more commonly speak of it, the indestructibility of matter. Their meeting was but a few years before Lavoisier fell a victim in the Revolution. In his *Glance at Hahnemann*, the doctor's young lawyer friend, Ernst von Brunnow, tells us further that Hahnemann was in correspondence with Lavoisier, as well as with Hufeland and other contemporary physicians. Dr. Wagner, the Medical Officer of Health in Dresden, also gave him scope for the study of forensic medicine. Later, the Municipal Council allowed Hahnemann to act as *locum tenens* when Dr. Wagner, owing to ill-health, had to withdraw from practice. The work of the Medical Officer was particularly strenuous, incidentally including being "willing to treat the wealthy citizens for a small consideration and the poor out of Christian charity." Of the nine heads defining the several branches of the responsibilities involved, section 3 alone decreed that he should treat and medically supervise the inmates of (i) the Military Hospital, (ii) the Workhouse, (iii) the Cross School, (iv) the Orphanage, (v) the Prisons.

It was no doubt in the discharge of the last-named duty that an insight was gained of a character which led Hahnemann later to become an ardent advocate of prison reform.

With a pen dipped in the indelible ink of an

exquisite sense of justice and compassion, he wrote in after years:

> "The civic crown merited by him who improves the prisons has been gained from us in Germany by an Englishman—Howard. Wagnitz followed in his steps. It is inconceivable how often the most destructive vapours are concentrated in these dens of misery. . . . I shall allude only to those where the imprisonment is for life, and to those gaols where prisoners guilty of capital crimes are kept until the termination of their trial (often for several years), the visitation and inspection of which is not infrequently the cause of infectious diseases.
>
> "Now, as in the true spirit of laws that are free from all barbarity, even the punishment of death should (and can have) no other aim than to render an incorrigible criminal innocuous and to remove him from human society, what else can both these kinds of imprisonment be for, except rendering the prisoner harmless, in the former case for life, in the latter for a certain time, pending the duration of trial? None but Syracusan tyrants could dream of uniting a more inhuman intention with such prisons."

After this Hahnemann pleads for structural changes, as for two windows opposite to each other, or, where this is impossible, "three windows to each small cell." Every fragment of his varied experience contributed something fresh and added to his qualifications. Not alone

FIRST PRACTICE AND MARRIAGE

in walking the hospitals or at the bedside of private patients did a physician such as he "qualify."

During Hahnemann's residence in Dresden the support of his family (with the exception of the twelve months' work as *locum tenens*) was maintained chiefly by literary work. Besides having completed the translation of Demachy's large work, he also translated two more by the same author, and a work by B. van den Sande on *Signs of the Purity and Adulteration of Drugs*, which was brought out jointly under both names by a Dresden publisher.

Besides this scientific output, Hahnemann had both translated and published the classic story of the great twelfth century theologian Abelard, who, whilst lecturing to his students in the Cathedral of Notre Dame, had within those precincts that other pupil, the Canon's niece, Heloise, destined to have a name forever bound up with his, though life forbade permanence to their union. We can easily imagine that a man of Hahnemann's idealism and experience in an almost completely satisfying marriage must have been keenly impressed by the poignancy of the grief that befell those sundered lovers. He it was who wrote later to a close and valued associate in his work: "Nothing in the world can replace the heavenly friendship that you miss in the absence of such a tie." The rendering of *Abelard and Heloise* into German, was, however, to be his only excursion into the sphere of classical romance, so wide was to be the range of his interest in the medical field, and so exacting the experimental labours which he required of himself in pursuit of knowledge.

When Dr. Wagner's illness ended in his death, Hahnemann applied for the post of Medical Officer of Health permanently, in spite of the exacting nature of its responsibilities. This, however, was given to an older man, and thus it is that we find him moving to Leipzig in September, 1789. There he would not find the courtly displays or the military functions that characterised the capital of the neighbouring state. These concerned the young doctor little, though he was in no way lacking in professional ambition. He was forcibly drawn to Leipzig by that spirit of learning which characterises a University town, and of which a University is the natural guardian. There too, were to be found those important people, the booksellers, and it is to this day a celebrated centre of book publication and sale.

In the year following this move we read of the death of his mother also, with whom Hahnemann appears to have had some estrangement. This, however, had happily been dispersed by now, as we can judge from a letter to the young doctor from his elder sister Charlotta, written in 1789. Charlotta, we are told, was Hahnemann's favourite sister, and her correspondence with her brother Samuel continued over a number of years. We can trace in it a Christian outlook of a profoundly evangelical character, reflecting probably the spirit which pervaded their early home, a lively interest in all that surrounded her life, and an education sufficient to merit her employment at one time as teacher in a nobleman's family.

In Leipzig the support of his now growing family was maintained chiefly by literary work, as had been the case in Dresden, except during the one year when he had undertaken duties for the Municipal Council. These years were no doubt those to which he refers later, when writing to Hufeland, as the period during which increasing dismay at the methods of treatment then current led him to withdraw from practice. Happily for Hahnemann, his growing reputation as an original thinker now led to his receiving valuable commissions from publishers. Prominent societies such as the "Leipzig Economical Society" and the "Academy of Science of the Electorate of Mayence" elected the doctor as an honorary member. When we realise that during his four years in Dresden he published more than 2,200 printed pages of matter, partly translations, partly original essays, etc., we can gauge something of the enthusiasm with which this son of Gottfried Hahnemann, with his one modest treatise on painting, laboured with his pen, in what has been described as his "fine, minute hand, beautiful and painstaking to the end of his days." We have a clue to the clearness of his small handwriting in the discovery that he wrote with an unsplit quill. These essays included an exposition of Hahnemann's "Wine test," which was subsequently adopted officially in Prussia. A letter from the Royal Prussian Police Directorate at this time recommended all in the wine trade "to have their present stock and their future supplies tested at once with Hahnemann's liquor." "He seems," observes a living writer, "to have been the first to discover that sulphuretted hydrogen in *acid* solution precipitates arsenic, lead, antimony, silver, mercury, copper, tin or bismuth, but not iron. Till this discovery there was no means of distinguishing readily iron from lead in solution, and wine dealers were often accused of adulterating wine with sugar-of-lead (a criminal offence) when the metal found was in reality iron."

Besides this there was yet another work on *"Poisoning by Arsenic: its treatment and forensic detection,"* from which the sphere of legal chemistry received new stimulus. As the result of his researches, Hahnemann demanded the restriction of the sale of this poison, which at that time was a constituent of popular "fever powders" sold by various tradesmen. It is significant that his suggestions for the prescribing of poison in general, which were afterwards given effect to, are still followed in detail to the present time. He further not only classified a great number of antidotes, but in giving his authorities from nearly four hundred authors, in various languages and of several centuries, he gave to each of his eight hundred and sixty-one passages quoted the exact reference as regards page and volume! We glimpse here the relentless thoroughness with which Hahnemann set himself to any task.

For forty years it was Hahnemann's custom to sit up the whole of one night out of four, working, translating, studying, writing. That he

FIRST PRACTICE AND MARRIAGE 65

lived to a ripe age, preserving a considerable measure of strength and health is indeed surprising, for, as he himself once observed, "Man (*i.e.* the delicate human machine) is not constituted for overwork."

The treatise on forensic medicine was offered "as the first fruits of the Author to His Majesty the good Kaiser Joseph."

lived to a ripe age, preserving a considerable
measure of strength and health is indeed surprising, for, as he himself once observed, "mankind, the delicate human machine, is not constructed for overwork."

The Ruolina ex torenze medicine was offered
as the first fruits of the Author to His Majesty
the good Kaiser Joseph."

CHAPTER IV

POVERTY AND GROWING RECOGNITION

Leipzig 1789-1792

It was in this Leipzig period that the first volume of Hahnemann's *Friend of Health* was produced, in which he appears as a searching commentator on hygienics. Of this work (and also of the *Handbook for Mothers*) Dr. Richard Haehl of Stuttgart writes: "Even to-day it is a real pleasure to read these entertaining and instructive essays. . . . Grave and forcible, even frankly indignant when need arises, yet full of humour and satire where the subject permits; at times chatting easily and cheerfully, and at others giving grave advice; using now the dialogue and now the letter form, entering into an instructive discussion with wonderful variety and most skilful and forcible use of language, Hahnemann turns to his readers in these works." In this suggestive summary of the author's style and manner of approach do we not almost feel we have met the man himself? The latter work, *i.e.* the *Handbook for Mothers*, was not Hahnemann's, but a translation from a French "abstract" from the writings of the great Rousseau which had been made by order of the National Convention in the second year of the French Republic. The book begins with a saying from Rousseau: "The earliest education is the most important. The education of man begins at his birth." Hahnemann no doubt now recognised the source of some of the most valued maxims learnt from his father, for Rousseau's influence, especially in matters relating to education, had for some years been spreading over Europe.

From 1789 to 1792 has been referred to as "the first Leipzig period," that is to say, the first since Hahnemann's marriage. Only part of it was spent in the city itself.

To live more easily within his means, with the five children already born to him, and to give these children a better chance of healthy growth, they removed to a little place, Stotteritz by name, situated to the south-east of the University town. It appears to have been a step with counter-balancing disadvantages. These indeed proved in the long run to more than outweigh any real gain, with the important exception of the purer atmosphere, of the value of which Hahnemann was duly aware.

In *Ecce Medicus*, by Dr. Burnett, we find a description of the doctor during his stay in the village: "He there clad himself in the garb of the very poor, wore clogs of wood and helped his wife in the house and kneaded bread with his own hands." It was also probably in Stötteritz that Hahnemann, after toiling all day long at his task of translating for the press, frequently assisted his courageous wife to wash the clothes at night, and as they were unable to purchase soap they employed raw potatoes for the purpose.

In the conversation between Socrates and Physon in the *Worth of Outward Show* (an original work of Hahnemann's written after the manner of a Platonic Dialogue) we find touches of thought and feeling revealing, it seems, Hahnemann's high valuation of his own family in these otherwise distressing times: "At what price wouldst thou part with thy five children?" Socrates asks Physon, who has but recently inherited a great fortune. "Certainly not for all my wealth. Physicians would be kings could they make women fruitful or save children from death." Socrates: "Thou art right, but in that case thy wife could not have been much less valued?" Physon: "By Juno, if she still lived I would not part with her for millions! That charming woman, with whose fidelity and thriftiness and goodness, and excellent manner of bringing up children when I used to live upon boiled beans, all the treasures of the earth are not to be compared." If this literary fragment from the doctor's pen is biographical at all, it certainly belongs to the period at which we have arrived—if we may judge by the number of Physon's offspring. The work closes with a portrayal of Hahnemann's "ideal physician." It may here be quoted, if only for its own intrinsic beauty.

"Knowest thou," says Socrates, "the man that has just passed us in a coarse woollen garment? In his venerable aged form beams universal philanthropy. That is Eumenes, the physician. The many thousands that he yearly makes by the practice of his art he does not spend in fine country houses and the other vain trifles of the luxurious. His happiness consists in doing good! About the tenth part of his large income he uses for his limited wants, the rest he puts out to interest in the State. And how? thou askest me. To the poor he gives his aid, his medical skill. With his stores he supports the convalescent families until they can again help themselves, and with the costliest of his wines he revives the dying. He seeks out the miserable in their dirty hovels and appears to them as a beneficent divinity; yes, when the all-vivifying sun, the image of the unknown God, refrains from showing the dying its life-bestowing face, and even at midnight, he appears in the huts of the miserable to assist them, and lavishes on them consolation, advice, and aid. They worship him as our ancestors worshipped the beneficent demi-gods, Osiris, Ceres and Æsculapius. Wilt thou soon commence to envy him? Go, Physon, and engage in some better pursuits, and then count on my esteem."

We shall not be far wrong, perhaps, if we trace some vivid personal experiences in these lines.

In a later essay entitled *The Prevention of Epidemics in General*, we certainly catch sight of the doctor on his rounds, amongst the sorriest members of society. In this work the psychological as well as the physical implications of the bad conditions prevailing in the poorest areas are imaginatively drawn with a remarkable realism, force and subtlety.

From amongst such passages we may take the following:

"But chiefly are the contagious pestilences in towns harboured, renewed, promoted and rendered more contagious and more murderous, in the small low houses situated close to the town walls, huddled together in narrow damp lanes or otherwise deprived of the access of fresh air, where poverty dwells, the mother of dirt, hunger and despondency. In order to save firing and the expensive rent, several miserable families are often packed close together, often all in one room, and they avoid opening a window or a door to admit fresh air, because the cold would enter along with it. He alone whose business takes him into these abodes of misery can know how the animal matters of the exhalation and of the breath are there concentrated, stagnant and putrefying; how the lungs of one are struggling to snatch from those of another the small quantity of vital air in the place, only to render it back laden with the effete matters of the blood; how the dim melancholy light from their small darkened windows is conjoined with the relaxing humidity and the mouldy stench of old rags and decayed straw; and how grief, envy, quarrelsomeness and other passions strive to rob the inmates of their little bit of health. In such places it is that infectious pestilences not only smoulder on easily and almost constantly when a spark falls upon them, but where they take their rise, burst forth and even become fatal to the wealthy citizens."

The fragment is splendidly crowned with the unwavering assertion: "It is the province of the authorities and the fathers of the country to change these birthplaces of pestilence into healthy happy human dwellings."

In a letter written soon after the family's migration to Stötteritz, we can actually witness the sway of the scales as Hahnemann puts the advantages or disadvantages into first one and then the other side, as regards this place of residence.

"If I were single or had not five children it would be different. But in any case, elsewhere my expenses would be heavier. Besides, I am so much my own master here. . . What I now earn, little as it is—more than suffices me! I cannot reckon much on income from practice. . . . I am too conscientious to prolong illness, or make it appear more dangerous than it really is. Pity, or love of peace, make me reticent in my claims—I am therefore constantly the loser and I can only look upon my practice as food for the heart."

In his work on "Poisoning by Arsenic," Hahnemann's disgust at the standards of medical practice with which a number of his professional colleagues were content, had already expressed itself in some scathing comments:

"A number of causes for several centuries reduced the dignity of that God-like science, practical medicine, to a wretched breadwinning, a glossing over of symptoms, a degrading commerce in prescriptions—God help us!—to a trade that mixes the disciples of Hippocrates with the riff-raff and medical rogues, in such a way that one is indistinguishable from the other."

The difficulties experienced at this time are even more clearly mirrored in another letter, dated August 29th, 1791, exactly a year to the day of the month after the previous one:

"It is impossible to live another year here in this village. I cannot subsist on literature alone; moreover, I have no suitable room for chemical work. I have to send for everything from the town by special messengers, except dry bread. I should have taken a house in Leipzig long ago, where I should like to live, had not famine, unhealthy air and high rents driven me out of the town for the sake of my sickly children; now that they are sturdy and strong, should I shut them up again in the town atmosphere of Leipzig with all its expenses? Life there means almost unsurmountable hardships, especially with a crowd of five small children. . . I would risk being criticised for wandering about the earth; it suffices that I undertake nothing without good reason. . . . I want a place where I can live quietly and privately, and yet can enlarge my knowledge as a scholar, surrounded by good people, and able to bring up my children straight and sensibly. My best friends in Leipzig would like to have me among them again; but they are too wealthy on the one hand to be able to understand my position, and on the other hand they cannot look at it with the eyes of a medical man."

In the same year, when the inevitability of some new venture had presented itself with unmistakable clearness, Hahnemann wrote to a Mining Director, in whose judgment he confided: "Are you able to give me good counsel concerning my change of abode? I am longing for it." Was this a friendship formed in Hettstedt?

This short move within the immediate neighbourhood of Leipzig proved to be the beginning of a series of seemingly aimless steps, a sequence of wanderings, over a number of years. Driven or drawn from one township to another, he accepted the dictates of circumstance, sometimes by reason of the need of fuller laboratory opportunities, at others because otherwise favourable conditions did not admit of earning sufficient, unless he practised against his principles, or, as instanced above, to reduce expenses and more especially to obtain healthy conditions for his family. Yet even these uncertainties and changes, with all the practical inconveniences involved, did not prevent a continuance of his activities. The nature of his work was, however, to become more and more of a literary and experimental character. Profoundly apprehensive of the harm that could be done in countless cases by resorting to the current medical methods,

GROWING RECOGNITION

Hahnemann in anguish and uncertainty of mind withdrew altogether or partially from their use.

In 1790 a treatise on *Materia Medica* by an Englishman, Cullen, was translated. The first edition of this had been published in London seventeen years earlier, followed by a second edition in two volumes the year before Hahnemann brought out his translation of it.

In the second volume of the work twenty pages were given up entirely to Peruvian Bark. This drug was known also as Cinchona Bark, because it had been the means of curing a Countess of Chinchon, whose husband was Viceroy of Peru, and through whom it was introduced into Europe, in 1640. This was indeed one of the most important of the drugs added to our pharmacopœia through the discovery of America. When the Countess brought back supplies of the bark to Spain, the priests immediately availed themselves of its curative powers, so much so that it also took on the name of Pulvis Jesuiticus We are told in that delightful book *The Mystery of the Art of the Apothecary* that whilst they charged the rich the price of its weight in gold, they gave it to the poor. It was not then suspected that its remarkable efficacy in curing fevers of various types would become the occasion of a series of experiments leading to the founding of an alternative School of Medicine, with its fully qualified medical advocates and hospitals throughout the civilised world. The *British Medical Journal* of December 30th, 1928, gave two whole pages to the extremely interesting history of the medicine, omitting, however, any reference to the part it played in initiating Hahnemann into a strenuous line of research.

"Whilst he was busy," writes Brunnow, "with a translation of the *Materia Medica* of Cullen, the celebrated English physician, he fell into such indignation at the confused attempts to explain the way in which cinchona suppresses ague, that he determined to cut the Gordian knot by making a trial of the medicine on his own body. No sooner thought than done. He took accordingly, at several times, strong doses of cinchona, such as the physicians of the day prescribed for the sick. How great was his astonishment when he found himself suffering from a strong paroxysm of ague! Then flashed on his mind the lucid thought, which gave him the key to all specific treatment. 'Does the cinchona bark,' he asked himself, 'which cures ague, produce the same?' Is the so-called specific curing power based on this principle? Does the same faculty of producing artificial diseases similar to those natural ones for which they are remedial, exist in all admitted specific medicines? He then tried a series of active substances, singly, on himself, and found his experiment confirmed by the corresponding results in each case. Every remedy of approved value brought on him, on trial, a disease similar to that for whose cure it was ordinarily given. He was also astonished at the great abundance of other symptoms, undreamed

GROWING RECOGNITION

of in the old Materia Medica, which these tried medicines presented to him. These hitherto unknown and peculiar effects of medicines inspired him with the hope of being able to cure many other diseases that had a characteristic similarity to the effects primarily produced. His theoretical presupposition was soon crowned with success."

These doses of cinchona produced not only the chief phenomena but minor symptoms which to a greater or lesser extent accompany malaria. He now "came face to face with the fact that this drug, which so surely and so often cured ague, was capable of producing in his own healthy body the phenomena of ague." . . . "This experiment," the writer continues, "was a ray of light to Hahnemann, for it suggested a possible clue to curative relations between drugs and cases of disease, a clue which he eagerly followed up." (We quote here from Dr. C. E. Wheeler's introduction to Hahnemann's *Organon of the Rational Art of Healing* in the "Everyman" Library.)

Even those who have accepted Hahnemann's finding on this occasion and his subsequent philosophy in medical practice, have differed in their explanation of the very distinct results obtained. One writer has supposed that Hahnemann must have previously been a victim of malaria, another that he had at least the malaria germ awaiting incubation in his constitution. There appears to be no evidence for the first supposition, nor any reason to assume that he was suffering from latent infection. Nor is there anything in our knowledge of Hahnemann's health to suggest that his was a physical temperament prone to that type of disorder.

A Berlin pharmacologist, Professor Lewin, covers the ground of "necessary conditions" much more satisfactorily, because his statements are based purely on experiment. Lewin, in his work *The Secondary Effects of Remedies*, speaking of "the much discussed and contested quinine fever," writes:

> "There is no doubt that for its manifestation it only requires a *special individuality*. With such a special tendency even very small quantities of cinchona, for instance, 0.06 gramme, produced this condition every time. . . . On the other hand, cases of quinine fever supervened where a debility of the body was absent. Therefore, the corresponding and frequently doubted observations of Hahnemann in himself, who after a large dose of cinchona bark was attacked by a cold fever similar to malaria, must be considered reliable."

Before the cinchona experiment Hahnemann had been impressed with the particular symptoms which mercury could produce, and had associated these with its healing capacities in syphilis. In this connection he had arrived at his very first faint intimations of "displacing a disease by similars," that is, by a medicine which could cause similar states to those which it could cure. Indeed, just because of the efficacious character of mercury in relation to that disease, Hahnemann had not only concentrated upon ascertaining the why and the wherefore of its good results, but had desired a still more excellent use of its healing properties. As a consequence of this research, he discovered a preparation of mercury for which the chemists had long been in quest, which was at the same time "very soluble and free from all corrosiveness." It is abundantly clear that Hahnemann was no theory seeker. He accepted willingly the laborious tasks imposed upon him by his questionings of Nature and the conclusions to which his observations led him.

Through his discovery of the power of cinchona (from which quinine is now derived) to produce the symptoms of malaria as well as to cure that disease, Hahnemann caught a glimpse of a *law of cure*, namely, that there was probably "no agent, no power in nature capable of morbidly affecting the healthy individual, which did not at the time possess the faculty of curing morbid states." In the words of Dr. John Clarke, cinchona bark was to Hahnemann what the falling apple was to Newton and the swinging lamp to Galileo. Hahnemann's translation of Cullen's work contained, amongst his annotations, a severe condemnation of various practices not only current, but often prosecuted with rigour by the physicians of his day. In one of these notes is to be found Hahnemann's first denunciation of venesection. "Bloodletting," he wrote scornfully, "fever remedies . . . and everlasting aperients and clysters form the circle in which the ordinary German physician turns round unceasingly." We can almost feel the pulse-beat of antagonism that such a declaration must, at least momentarily, have stirred throughout the profession. Yet it was not in the spirit of a mere challenge to controversy that these lines were penned. When suffering in countless cases was being needlessly increased, and the very aid upon which hope was fixed was turned to an instrument of defeat, Hahnemann felt that silence was impossible. Happily there were a few open-minded men like Hufeland who "could reconcile himself very well to Hahnemann's criticisms, which he recognised to be both justified and well-intentioned." Hufeland has been described as "one of the great philanthropic physicians who are true friends of the human race." He was alike friend and physician to Goethe, Schiller, and Herder. The most important of the four medical journals for which he was responsible bore his own name, "Hufeland's Journal," and this continually opened its columns to the writings of Hahnemann. Yet even Hufeland regarded Hahnemann's total rejection of venesection as "a sin of omission." There were, no doubt, excellent men, such as he, who were convinced that Hahnemann was wrong, and who used this method with the utmost caution, and only in specialised circumstances. But when one realises the widespread character of the practice of opening the veins of sick persons and the recklessness engendered by frequent recourse to it, the insufferable plight of innumerable patients, already at the lowest ebb in strength, can be imagined. Venesection indeed had its ruthless practitioners. Broussais, who was first an Army surgeon and then in 1820 and onwards chief Professor at the Hôpital Militaire d'Instruction in Paris, won for himself the name of "the medical Robespierre." A Greek physician commenting on his achievements observed, "Ibrahim Pasha has not killed so many men here as Broussais' system." Broussais' methods, we are told, "became fashionable."

In 1792 a calamity of public import led Hahnemann to a yet more vehement protest against this medical practice. The occasion lay in the grave illness of Emperor Leopold II of Austria, the brother of Marie Antoinette. This monarch, by various parties in Europe, was being looked to as a possible instrument in the maintaining of peace between Germany and France, which was still in the throes of revolutionary experience. Others, it is true, suspected Leopold of having entered into some agreement with Prussia against France. He had at least to his credit that he succeeded in pacifying Hungary and the Netherlands. In the present crisis much needed to be done, France at the moment being enraged at the sheltering of French refugees by the Germans. This was in the year preceding Victor Hugo's "Ninety-Three," when to have handed back these French nationals would almost assuredly have been to hand them over to the guillotine. Whether Leopold would have been helpful in this situation by a wise strategy, will never be known. Hopes and fears cherished in his direction were alike stunned by the announcement that he was dead. So unanticipated was this that suspicions of a political betrayal were not lacking.

But it was not in that sphere that an explanation of the event had to be sought. To meet the agitated curiosity of both sides a medical bulletin had to be published in Vienna. So superficial was this report in the eyes of Hahnemann, and so grave in its admissions, that he at once wrote a severe criticism of it in the *Anzeiger*, appending to it his full signature. In this he pointed out that the Emperor's doctor, Lagusius, had admittedly tried to fight the severe fever and its accompanying symptoms by venesection, and when this "failed to give relief" he proceeded to open the veins again and yet again, until blood-letting had been resorted to for a fourth time. "We ask," wrote Hahnemann, dismayed at this horrible confession of impotence, "from a scientific point of view, according to what principle has anyone the right to order a second venesection when the first has failed to bring relief? As for a third, Heaven help us; but to draw blood a fourth time when the three previous attempts failed to alleviate! To abstract the fluid of life four times in twenty-four hours from a man who has lost flesh from mental overwork, combined with a long continued diarrhœa, without procuring any improvement —Science pales before this." In the bulletin not only had venesection been mentioned, but also the use of "other means," a term sufficiently indeterminate in a public announcement of such gravity as to lead Hahnemann to exclaim in his response: "Germany—Europe—has a right to ask by *what* means?"

The doctors responsible were then challenged to give public justification for such a line of treatment, which so completely robbed the patient of his sparse reserves of strength essential for the combating of the disease. A more complete bulletin was promised by the physician-in-ordinary, but it was never forthcoming. Bitter attacks on Hahnemann, alternating with protestations of appreciation of his courage in exposing the interior significance of the treatment that had been meted out to the unfortunate monarch, followed one another in the pages of the *Anzeiger*. One of his supporters, a medical man, wrote: "Why should a learned man who is in a position to speak, fail to do so? Is not such a far-seeing, unprejudiced, cool and disinterested observer a representative, or rather a precursor of posterity. He is what the morning star is to the sun."

"Far-seeing," "unprejudiced" and "disinterested": in the selection of these adjectives Hahnemann's defender was well guided, but we can hardly believe that Samuel Hahnemann in his expression of condemnation at the methods that had been employed in this case could be said to be "cool." Zeal such as his by virtue of its very nature was, one would suppose, at least warm. And it must be remembered that we have here a man who could fight other battles than those of Emperors and Princes. He it was who left it on record that the best prepared and the purest medicine should be used by a physician even for "the meanest slave, for he, too, is a man." There is also a suggestive postscript in Hahnemann's letter to one of the princes, who had asked his advice on the choice of a family physician. It reads: "One word more! Before you finally fix on him, see how he behaves to the poor, and if he occupies himself at home with some useful work."

On the side of destructive criticism Hahnemann had now entered the lists, with all but a few of the whole army of his professional colleagues arrayed against him. Little at this time did he realise that when this battle had been waged, yet another, on the side of his constructive contribution to medical science and art, awaited him.

CHAPTER V

HAHNEMANN AS PHYSICIAN OF THE MENTALLY DISORDERED

Georgenthal 1792-1793

THE study of mental disorders, in the days of which we are speaking, had few specialists. Yet better ideas on the treatment of the insane were astir in various places.

In 1792 the Duke Ernst von Sachsen-Gotha, having heard of the good reputation of Samuel Hahnemann as a physician, and of his intention to devote himself to this kind of work, placed a wing of his hunting castle at his disposal. This was four years before William Tuke, the English Quaker, had finally established the Retreat in York—he had conceived the project in 1791—and a year before Pinel reformed the Bicêtre Asylum in Paris. Each of these three reformers appears to have worked independently.

Being now provided with an opportunity of treating the insane under ideal conditions, Hahnemann revealed the fact that for several years previously he had made a special study of "diseases of the most lingering and hopeless nature generally, and of hypochondria and insanity in particular."

Publicity was given to his wish to serve these

unfortunate patients. This was done jointly with Councillor Becker, of Gotha, who was both a personal friend and the editor of the paper called *The Anzeiger*. It will be remembered that this was the journal which had opened its columns to Hahnemann's protest against the treatment of Joseph II of Austria.

The announcement appeared on February 6th of the above year, under the heading "Proposal for a much-needed relief Institution for Mental Patients of the better classes." Yet, in spite of the clear intention to restrict the use of the benevolent Prince's castle to persons of what is called good social standing, it is interesting to note that the document breaks out compassionately into a plea for a rational treatment of the countless victims of insanity who were kept in confinement in the asylums run "in connection with prisons and workhouses." The appeal bears only the name of Becker, but it is not difficult to recognise Hahnemann's pen in those passages which show the mark of his experience.

"There is usually," it states, "only one doctor in charge of such an institution, although twenty would be required for the ultimate purpose of curing this large number of unfortunate inmates. Often a physician in such a position has neither the courage nor sufficient knowledge for this special branch of work." "These noblest of all creatures," it continues, "destined for the exalted use of reason, are here treated as wild beasts from Africa intended for exhibition would not be treated, or they are kept like inanimate objects for three, four, ten, thirty or more years—without contributing to the alleviation of their disease, without restoring them to the usefulness for which, in their former days, they had been so deserving of honour; they are kept, I say, with an indolence which does no credit to our century. This is inflicted upon the middle and lower classes of the population. 'They must rest content with the existing institutions,' says the heartless onlooker."

The dilemma of distinguished persons who have no alternative to such places into which to place their mentally broken relatives is then described. We can later recognise Councillor Becker's part in the following sentences:

"I need not add more, I think, in order to make you feel how desirable it would be to have a decent home for this class of patient. I am glad to be able to announce that a proposition in this spirit has been made by a physician who is both scientific and practical, and who is well known to me and to the scientific world. He is taking steps to establish an institution which will accommodate about four better-class mental patients. . . . They will neither be beaten nor confined in chains, and no harsh treatment will be used in order to bring them back to reason."

In August this notice was followed by another:

"The Nursing Home for mental patients . . . has now been open for some time. . . .

The first experiment which has already been made gives hope of happy results.

"The locality, where the home has come into existence through the generous help of the Sovereign, is Georgenthal, an important village with a law court and office for forestry. It is situated in one of the most beautiful districts at the foot of the Thüringerwald, three hours' journey from the capital Gotha. . ."

The patient referred to was one who had been recommended for treatment by the Duke himself, Klockenbring by name. This man was an author of highly susceptible disposition, having become insane through a malicious attack made on him, apparently with no justification, by a poet. His family physician in Hanover, together with others, had done all in his power to cure the patient. Alas, in vain! Even though there was a clear interval at times, the fury of the illness was soon redoubled.

These circumstances of the case are given by the author of *A Remarkable German, Klockenbring*. "About this time," the writer continues, "the famous Dr. Hahnemann, then residing in Gotha, made it known that he intended to dedicate all his time and all his capabilities to patients with diseases of the mind." The record goes on to state that after many enquiries there was only one opinion of this doctor, and that in June of 1792 Klockenbring was brought with a suitable escort to Georgenthal. It then goes on to quote from Hahnemann's own notes on the patient's fits of mania: "Incessantly, day and night, he kept on raving and was never composed for a quarter of an hour at a time. At one minute he spoke as a judge and delivered sentence; at another he would recite as Agamemnon. . . . Nothing was ever quite completed, but the new idea displaced the former with violent haste"; and again: "He smashed anything that came to hand at that period, even his piano, and then he put it together again in a peculiar manner in order, as he said, to find a complementary note."

For the first weeks Hahnemann simply observed the patient without giving him any medical treatment. Until February of the following year he then treated him both psychically and by medicine, and by that time was able to report to Klockenbring's wife that he was restored. As proof of this Klockenbring made a translation of a book by an Englishman, Arthur Young, on *State Economy in England*, and he was again able to take up remunerative work. There was, moreover, no relapse, though Klockenbring's death two years after his discharge was preceded by a period of apathy.

A criticism was levelled at Hahnemann by some of his contemporaries, because in this case he had asked a fee of a thousand thalers. When it is recollected that Klockenbring was a wealthy man, and that Hahnemann had given up the whole of several months to the one patient, it will be apparent that the criticism was an ungenerous one. In the doctor we find a man who was willing to work for either nothing, little, or much, according to the exigencies of the situation.

Besides Hahnemann's application for the ill-paid, though heavy, post of Medical Officer in Dresden, we have other instances of his willingness to ignore the winning of financial rewards when to have done so would have jeopardised his integrity as a physician or his freedom for research. More than once we have already seen him withdrawing entirely or almost entirely from practice because of his profound mistrust of the prevalent medical methods, for which he had so far found no alternative. And again, we have a delightful fragment of biography referring to later years given by Franz Hartmann, one of Hahnemann's disciples, in a work which appeared in 1844. Here he tells us that "year in, year out, Hahnemann treated twelve poor patients without a fee. They came at the same consulting hours and enjoyed the same rights as rich patients. For they were always taken in their turn, and no rich man was able to boast that he had received preference over the poor."

The view that his terms were too high had quite definitely an adverse effect on his work, for it appears that more than one application fell through on this ground. "I can well see that in Germany they are unable to appreciate efforts to cure an insane person," the doctor wrote to Counsellor Becker.

"How can anyone expect a physician to face the danger which is always present in mental cases, or expect that the careful active and passive precautions necessary for the safe-keeping of such as are devoid of reason, or that the time spent, the expensive upkeep of the nurses, the selection of the medicine, etc., should all be undertaken for a trifling sum—without even thinking of the gloominess of such work? Indeed, I should not like to undertake so much for a very small stipend. Therefore I share your opinion that I am justified in asking my rightful fees.

"Do come and see me soon. We are at present in great disorder on account of the building alterations, but I am quite able to spend a few hours with a good friend, and especially with you. . . ."

"Does one not wish, for one's own sake, to remunerate the diver more liberally than the man who walks down a few steps in safety?" This question in the same letter is characteristic of the doctor's attitude to the need "of a just return" throughout his life. Both from the preliminary announcement in the press and from the satisfactory results in the case cited, we can gather that Hahnemann had no idea of insanity as being incurable, though he stressed that it might become so through wrong treatment. In those days it was generally assumed not to be curable, an assumption attacked also by Pinel as "a prejudice injurious to humanity."

The cure of the mentally disordered, Hahnemann believed, was to be accomplished partly by psychological means, partly by dealing with the physical basis of life through medicines. Indeed, in his laborious search through the medical records of past generations and other lands he had not, we know, missed the illustration to the operation of the *law of similars* in medicine selection afforded in the cure by Hippocrates of his friend's mania by the use of hellebore, the properties of which plant if taken in sufficiently dangerous strength by those who are well can produce the symptoms of mania. Hahnemann recognised also certain diseases of the disposition which "with but slight implication of the body, originate and endure from emotional causes, such as continued anxiety, worry, vexation and exposure to terror or fright." For these he prescribed purely "psychical means" of cure. As regards the general manner of treatment, Hahnemann's writings offer a comprehensive though brief survey. It appears in an "Author's Note" to Section 198 of the *Organon*, and includes the following emphatic instructions:

> "Destructive acts and injuries must be prevented without reproaches to the patient, and everything must be arranged to prevent corporal punishment. For, as in mental disorders there can be no sense of wrong doing, so by all human justice there should be no punishments. Contradictions, eager explanations, violent corrections and harshness are as disastrous to the mind and soul of such patients as timid yielding at the wrong time. Above all, contempt, deceit and fraud exasperate these patients and aggravate their condition.

A semblance must always be maintained of treating them as reasonable beings."

A passage relating to the use of "suitable homœopathic remedies" shows that this was written after his formulation of a philosophy of medicine both as regards physical and psychological conditions. Yet although penned years after, through these lines we may picture the doctor at his difficult task in the hunting castle at Georgenthal, trying through a rational attitude to overcome his patient's disorder of mind.

Haehl, commenting on these psychological effects of medicines homœopathically prescribed, states that Hahnemann as a matter of fact acquired a knowledge of psychiatry (science of mental disorder) greater than that of Pinel. Whereas both upheld the cause of humane treatment for mental patients, Hahnemann in addition laid the foundations of a medicinal treatment of mental illness. "The Creator of medicinal virtues," he wrote, "has had particular regard to this important feature of disease, namely, alterations in the mental and moral condition." Every medicine "proved" by Hahnemann before he wrote this had revealed its mental symptoms.

Had other patients followed, it is clear that Hahnemann would have continued to throw the whole weight of his research into similar experiments, both for the purpose of curing individuals and for bequeathing to others the results of his experience in this kind of practice.

Happily, circumstances prevented specialisation in the cure of insanity. One factor was, probably, an inability in Hahnemann to deport himself quite as others, and to do just those things expected by a "patron" however benevolent. Thus, what proved afterwards to be his life work, with its precise contribution to psychiatry as well as to general medicine, was not missed by his remaining too long in this sphere, as it might otherwise have been. Hahnemann's notes on Klockenbring's case end with the reflection: "However wearing, even when followed by success, the uninterrupted and personal attention given to this kind of patient may be, seeing that it is capable of killing the joy of life more effectually than anything else and sadly shakes the soul of the humane and thoughtful physician, yet I feel strongly the call to continue the work. . . ." This document bears the postscript, "In my garden in Brunswick." We find also an interesting postscript to a letter written only a year after, showing his sustained interest in the whole question: "I read yesterday a story like Klockenbring's in an old book that appealed to me very much. In 'Boneti medicina septentrionalis fol. Pars 1, 200-204.' When you can do so, read it! It has always been the same in the world, even 130 years ago."

In a private house later on the difficulties of such work were great. Yet even this was attempted. In one case Hahnemann's refusal to take in a mental case sent without due warning was explained thus: "You know how careful I am on this point, and have to be, on account of a lot of little children who can be easily injured." Yet although Hahnemann made the attempt of carrying out treatment in his home which he describes as "a really pretty, comfortable and also favourable house," it proved more than he could undertake. Through the appearance of an unexpected trait of violence, the plan of keeping one of his patients until cured had to be abandoned. Before so doing Hahnemann, it appears, had approached at least ten different persons with a view to obtaining their help as attendants. And this with the offer of generous remuneration, but all to no effect!

This concern for the mentally disordered began, as we know, several years before the hunting castle experiment. From a letter addressed from Mölln and dated September 20th, 1800, we can see that it also persisted for a considerable number of years following it.

In Singer's *Short History of Medicine* we read that "while Pinel was beginning the humaner treatment of insanity in France, considerable interest was aroused in the subject in Germany." The writer then adds: "There, however, the medical profession was still under the influence of Stahl, who regarded all forms of insanity as perversions of the moral tendencies of the soul produced by sin." The author appears in his survey to have missed a notable exception in this Saxon doctor.

It may have been noticed that for some time Hahnemann had only "observed" his patient. In his essay *The Medicine of Experience*, we find recurrent references to the need of exact and sensitive powers of observing, and analogies are drawn from the sphere of draughtsmanship. This reminds us that Hahnemann grew up in an artist's household, and was no doubt a witness of those attainments in drawing in the faithful reproductions of plant forms, whether from copies or from nature, which characterise porcelain designs. Thus he writes as regards obtaining an adequate account of the pathological condition of a patient (in order to prescribe with equal precision): "To trace the picture of the disease, the physician requires to proceed in a very simple manner. All that he needs is carefulness in observing and fidelity in copying." For the cultivation of powers of observation he gives various instructions.

Elsewhere we read:
"To educate us for the acquirement of this faculty, an acquaintance with the best writings of the Greeks and Romans is useful, in order to enable us to attain directness in thinking and in feeling; as also appropriateness and simplicity in expressing sensations and the art of drawing from nature, as it sharpens and practises our eye, and thereby also our other senses, teaching us to form a true conception of objects, and to represent what we observe, truly and purely, without any addition from the fancy. A knowledge of mathematics also gives us the requisite severity in forming a judgment."

So much for Hahnemann's plea for a truth sharpened into a fine accuracy. Of the spirit in which the physician is to pursue this work he also reveals his conception:

> "He knows," Hahnemann writes, "that observations of medical subjects must be made in a sincere and holy spirit, as if under the eye of the all-seeing God, the Judge of our secret thoughts, and must be recorded so as to satisfy an upright conscience, in order that they may be communicated to the world, in the consciousness that no earthly good is more worthy of our zealous exertions than the preservation of the life and health of our fellow creatures."

Such expressions are reminiscent of the spirit of the Hippocratic oath, with which Hahnemann was undoubtedly acquainted.

That Samuel Hahnemann himself drew, we know, for, apart from the mathematical and mechanical sketches reproduced in the biography by Haehl and the "rebus" which hangs in the tavern at Meissen, it is impossible to imagine him advising others to adopt a method of improving their powers which he had not himself utilised.

In a delightful Presidential Address delivered to the Bristol Medico-Chirurgical Society on "The Debt of Medicine to the Fine Arts," Dr. J. A. Nixon says:

> "The Greeks of the fifth century B.C. were distinguished by intellectual acuteness and artistic gifts, a fertile combination for the

growth of science. . . . 'Progress was at last made in the art of medicine because the physicians of Greece shared with her poets and sculptors the same splendid faculties of keen sight and faithful reproduction of things seen. . . .' As we read the Hippocratic writings we realise that the acuity of observation that Praxiteles and Pheidias brought to their masterpieces of sculpture finds expression in the Hippocratic description of clinical cases."

Whilst we may not be able to agree with Dr. Nixon when he says later that "the theories of Hippocrates were admittedly as speculative and erroneous as any" (members of the Hippocratic School at least appear to have anticipated the use of "the law of similars" in medicine, and, in surgery, the treatment of blindness, without visible ocular disease, by the so-called modern method of craniectomy), we can follow him again when he says that whenever Hippocrates confined himself to the simple observation of patients and their behaviour, the artistic perception broke forth as in his inimitable description of the countenance of the dead person. For is not simplicity in observing the foundation of truth in all the arts, whether literary or plastic? "Hippocrates," he continues, "had the good fortune to be living in the age of Pericles, one of those rare epochs when artists, philosophers, and men of action cease to live in isolation, but breathe a common air and catch light and heat from each other's thoughts."

Hahnemann, alas, was not so fortunate in his

contemporaries, but it seems that where circumstances failed him, he filled in the lack by an extension of his sympathies and understanding into realms of interest which lay around the particular province of his own choice. From the past he wrested its profoundest ideals in thought—the teachings of the Greek philosopher Plato and the Chinese seer Confucius alike rejoiced him; such names amongst painters as Michael Angelo, Raphael, and Titian he held in honour, whilst from the present he drew the widest opportunities for an unfeigned search for what was true and beneficent for his fellows. It is true to say that Christian Samuel Hahnemann not only made his own work, but also in a large measure his own world.

CHAPTER VI

THE APOTHECARIES' LEXICON AND THE FRIEND OF HEALTH—PART II

Molschleben, Göttingen, Pyrmont, Wolfenbüttel, Brunswick, 1793-1796

HAHNEMANN still travelled from point to point, the villages or townships in which he lived for more or less brief periods hanging like beads upon a thread of nomadic experience seemingly fruitless, yet moving forward to an assured goal. Molschleben, Göttingen, Pyrmont, Wolfenbüttel and Brunswick were all dwelt in between 1793 and 1796. Hamburg at one point had to be abandoned, for its high standard of living would assuredly have "swallowed him up." Nor had travelling in those days its present conveniences, whilst it appears to have had at least in measure some of the perils known to us. A letter from Hahnemann, in the year 1794, records one serious misadventure:

"I have stuck here at Göttingen and shall probably not get any further, but stay here. The upsetting of the carriage at Mulhausen, of which you have probably heard, and in which we nearly lost our lives (to heal our wounds we had to remain nearly eight days at Mulhausen), has shattered my wife's health so much, and the children have become so afraid of driving, that it is becoming impossible for me to come any further—at least without probable danger to my family in general, and especially to the suckling baby boy. The driver who overturned us is one of the most careless and dangerous men I have ever known. I hope no one else will suffer through him."

Of the conditions under which the family travelled we get a glimpse in an undated letter:

"I should be very glad if I could find out through you how much a driver with four horses and a very roomy carriage requires a day, without my having to trouble about fodder. If I can agree with the man and like the carriage, which I do not know beforehand, and if the cost for the day is reasonable, I might (if I wish) use him until I get there. But I cannot decide on a definite length of road nor define the number of days. It must be understood that in any case his return does not concern me. On an average I drive not more than 20 to 25 miles a day, and I decide my plans each day in order to be free to make just such a short journey as I like."

We have an amusing description of his arrival at Göttingen in "a kind of emigrant's carriage with his numerous family."

At Göttingen a certain Dr. Pfaff, who met him at his work in the Lying-in Hospital, observed that the doctor, whom he calls "the then famous Hahnemann," gave the impression of being a

Herrnhuter and a mystic. His mysticism apparently betrayed itself chiefly in the habit he had of always having some of the shutters down in his front room. By a "Herrnhuter" we may understand Dr. Pfaff wished to convey the demeanour of a grave and inward-minded man, such as belonged to the (Moravian) Community bearing that name.

That there was a touch of mysticism—deeper even than that implied by closed shutters!—many of Hahnemann's pronouncements concerning the Creative Mind suggest.

> "The ever-beneficent Godhead animating the infinite universe," he wrote to a medical colleague, "dwells in us also, and gives us our faculty of reason as the highest, inestimable endowment, whilst from the fullness of His own moral character He implants in our conscience a spark of holiness. . . . Even when we depart this life, the great, unique and infinite Being, who suffuses happiness into all men, will continue to instruct us how to approach His perfect blessedness by further acts of goodness and to become more like Him to all eternity."

Such expressions are not unworthy to be placed side by side with those of such writers as the great eighteenth century Doctor of Divinity and mystic, William Law, who also wrote: "That this form of a Divine Life is in every man, and that no man is without witness of God in himself, is a truth as evident as anything that can be affirmed of human nature."

Yet Hahnemann, despite his profound sense of a universal and beneficent Deity, shrank from any metaphysical wrappings to truth. Indeed, we can well imagine him, like William Blake, exclaiming: "Alas for Mystery who never loosed her captives!" In a letter to his friend von Villers he revealed this attitude:

"I had known for some time that you had made our Kant available in France, but had not considered what an enormous effort it must have cost you to understand even his *Critique of Pure Reason*, as so many German-born scientists cannot fathom or understand Kant, let alone translate him into a language which is hardly capable of reproducing his modes of expression. This has been done for the good of mankind.

"I admire Kant very much, particularly because he draws the line of philosophy, and of all human knowledge, where experience ends. If the remaining part of what he has thought and written had only unfolded itself a little more clearly before the inner vision, I think that he would not have enveloped himself in a cloud of such obscure sentences. His whole accepted philosophy ought, I think, to have been easily understood at least by all educated people, and to have been so comprehensible that no misunderstanding could arise. It is, however, only my humble self that thinks this, and perhaps I am wrong. It is for this reason that I only value Plato when he is quite comprehensible and speaks clearly.

If the so-called philosophers who followed Kant had not written even more mystically and allowed their imagination so much play, if, in one word, they had kept, as Kant wanted them to, within the boundaries of experience, my fight to-day for the reform of medical science would have been an easier one."

Dr. Pfaff, referring to the occasions on which they met, says:

"I called on him several times and he did not then say anything about homœopathy, but expected to cure through the chemical properties of medicines. One of his children sickened with dysentery, and Hahnemann hoped to fight the enemy through the antiseptic properties of charcoal; but the illness became worse, and . . . he gave the small patient over to me and happily I cured him."

The value of this brief glance at Samuel Hahnemann through Dr. Pfaff in this year is that it shows us that four years after the translating of Cullen's treatise on Materia Medica he was still uncommitted in any final way to the Law of Similars in the selection of his remedies, nor had the dynamization of medicines been carried to any length. Nor was Hahnemann yet under any concern, apparently, to expatiate to this obviously sympathetic physician, Dr. Pfaff, upon the philosophy of medicine that was forming in his own mind. For six years following the cinchona experiment Hahnemann remained silent as to his "findings." This deliberation is in accord with all that we can ascertain of the man's character. What he scorned in the methods adopted by others, the glossing over of ignorance with elaborate and often obscure theories, Hahnemann had no desire to tolerate in his own contribution to medical thought and practice. Nor can we at any point detect him thinking or working along one line exclusively, as his various activities show.

In connection with his early translation of Demachy's work, Hahnemann is referred to as one who without specialised tuition in chemistry or practical work in a chemical laboratory, was "often able to correct and supplement the Parisian chemist." That was in the year 1785, and now, in 1793, came a work of much greater importance from Hahnemann's pen, the *Apothecaries' Lexicon*. This appeared in four volumes. It could still be said that no laboratory experience, as we understand it, had fallen to his lot, except for his early experiments with his father-in-law in Dessau. Yet at every halting point, besides original contributions on the subject, translations of works from the French, English, Italian and other languages were forthcoming, and it is impossible to disassociate Hahnemann from intensive experiment. Too many of his works bear the impress of this. In Stötteritz we heard him lamenting that he had "no suitable room for such work," yet even under those unpropitious circumstances the work was continued. There was undoubtedly an unbroken chain of practical enquiries into chemical laws during the years that followed.

THE APOTHECARIES' LEXICON

The book now in question met with an appreciative reception from recognised quarters. In Crell's *Annals* at this time he is mentioned as "this famous analytical chemist." The reviewer in the *Medizinisch-Chirurgische Zeitung* stressed that "not only the apothecary but the physician also would be well advised to become familiar with it." From a professor in Erfurt further commendation was forthcoming from the outset. He wrote of the *Lexicon*, after seeing the first volume, as "an excellent work which every apothecary ought to procure—brevity, lucidity, decision and yet a completeness" distinguishing the work from all others of a similar character, adding that an examination of the work revealed much new and important matter.

During these years the second part of *The Friend of Health* appeared. Commenced in Leipzig it remains a record of the insight gained immediately before as a Medical Officer of Health in Dresden. This had by now been supplemented by his experiences as an ordinary practitioner treating the inhabitants, both of rich and of poor neighbourhoods. Of the tragedies of the latter, as we have already shown, few could have proved more sensitive or understanding observers. More, indeed, than an observer must this physician be called. Of their needs he became an advocate, combining in his advocacy ardour and fidelity to fact. In an article, "Things that spoil the air," included under the above general title, we gain a further glimpse into the underworld of suffering into which his work took him:

"Poverty," he writes, "has brought many injurious habits into this world, one of the worst of which is that where persons in the lower ranks of life, especially women, sit over a vessel filled with red-hot charcoal, in order thereby to save themselves the expense of a stove in winter. The closer the room is shut up in such circumstances, the more the external air is excluded, the more dangerous and fatal is this habit, for the air inside will soon become a stupefying poison.

"We feel an oppressive, stupefying headache, that seems to bore through both temples, at the same time we experience an inclination to vomit, which, however, is soon suppressed by a rapidly increasing comatose state, in which we sink helplessly to the ground and generally die without convulsions.

"When the person falls down, the clothes are apt to catch fire from the burning charcoal, and, indeed, fires have often originated in this manner, which are all the more dangerous because it is only when they have fairly burst forth that they will be observed by strangers, seeing that the person who originates them is too stupefied to extinguish the first flames."

It may be noted here that the folly is ascribed to privation—there is no word of censure. It is significant too that Hahnemann falls into the first person plural in one portion of his description —I am reminded by this of the American Quaker, John Woolman, who, forgetting his own name, became identified in a vision with the miners. Less impersonal is the language in the same article where greater follies—greater because without the plea of necessity—are noted in higher ranks of society. With a vivacity and truth not unworthy of some of our early novelists the passage further gives us an amusing scene of contemporary life.

"People who wish to be very genteel love to burn in the evening more candles than are necessary; and if they are entertaining company, they light up chandeliers, sconces and all other receptacles for candles they may possess, in order that the fashionably dressed ladies and gentlemen may see each other well. It is considered a capital holiday spectacle to see so many candles burning at once; it dazzles the eyes so brilliantly that we scarcely know where we are; it also costs a good round sum.

"But if we view all this display of candles in the proper light, we shall find that they spoil the air in a very ugly manner. Considering that they are only lighted for a number of guests who are to be well feasted, who, seated in rows pollute the atmosphere for each other by their breathing and exhalations, in a word, that they are only lighted for feasts and balls, . . . I know not what sort of complimentary speech I can make to my entertainer for purposely depriving me of the little bit of God's pure air, and giving me the very worst sort instead. . . . Amid how many attacks of faintness will not yon lady express her thanks to him, after having worked away for hours at her toilette preparing for the festivities, in the endeavour to diminish by one third the capacity of her chest by means of a whalebone apparatus, until, drawn in so tightly as to look like a wasp, she could scarcely take in air enough in a pure atmosphere: relish it who may, I must say for my part I have no wish to be regaled with so many candles in a room."

The wide range of his opportunities for observation is swiftly indicated in the few pages of this essay alone. We follow the doctor on his visits to homes where persons sleep where green fruit is stored and to where families dwell in rooms that are also store-rooms, "where domestic articles and food from the animal and vegetable kingdoms are kept in quantity, such as oils, candles, lard, raw, boiled or roasted meat, etc." Such are, needless to say, condemned as unhealthy.

From cellars we pass to houses where thick-leaved trees stand close to the windows hindering the entrance of light and spoiling the air by their exhalations at night, though "trees at a distance of from ten to twelve paces," Hahnemann tells us, "cannot be sufficiently recommended, as well on account of their beautiful appearance and their pleasant shade, as on account of the wholesomeness of their exhalations by day." The ignorance of the poor (as well as their misfortune) is also touched upon, and the short work ends with the characteristic question:

"Where is the compassionate man who will teach them something better?"

Hahnemann in his writings on epidemics touched on almost every aspect of the subject. He urged isolation hospitals and the most scrupulous cleanliness and care in three essays under the respective titles of *Protection against Infection in Epidemic Diseases; Plans for Eradicating a Malignant Fever;* and *Suggestions for the Prevention of Epidemics in General.* Anyone reading his works on hygiene could not but feel that Christian Samuel Hahnemann, like Bentham, made a sustained attempt "to draw a parallel between the physical and social sciences," and like that great Englishman, whose German contemporary he was, made a vital plea for an awakened and informed conscience on all matters touching Public Health. Truly Hahnemann was no man of one idea exaggerated out of all proportion to the scheme of things to which it belonged. The elimination of the cause where possible, including the abandonment of wrong ways of living, personal hygiene and medicinal treatment with appropriate accessory means, all found a place in his philosophy and practice.

We find also that Hahnemann was both acquainted with and concerned about a variety of factories and workshops. He writes:

> "In large *manufactories* and *workhouses* where the workpeople live in the house, those who fall ill should, whenever they commence to complain, be immediately separated from the healthy workmen, and kept apart until they

have completely recovered their health. . . . Great care should be taken always, but especially when disease is about, to have the workrooms and warerooms well aired and clean."

The essay previously quoted contains the crisp observation: "Six busy watchmakers do not spoil the air nearly so much as two workmen engaged in sawing wood." Again the tone of autobiography marks his style, and we seem almost to see the industrious watchmakers pause for a few moments to talk with the lively and kindly doctor of not yet thirty years, as he enters their workroom.

His personal attitude to those of his patients who had to work hard for their living is revealed in a letter to a tailor in Gotha:

"Man (that delicate human machine) is not constituted for overwork. If he does so from ambition, love of gain, or other praiseworthy or blameworthy motive, he sets himself in opposition to the order of nature, and his body suffers injury or destruction. The more so if his body is already in a weakened condition; then, what you cannot accomplish in a week you can do in two weeks. Your customers may not be willing to wait, but they cannot reasonably expect that you will make yourself ill and work yourself into the grave for their sake, leaving your wife a widow and your children orphans. It is not only the greater bodily exertion that injures you, but even more the attendant strain on the mind; the overwrought mind in its turn affects the body injuriously.

If you do not assume an attitude of calm indifference, adopting the principle of living first for yourself and only secondly for others, then there is small chance of your recovery. When you are in the grave, men will still be clothed, perhaps not so tastefully, but still tolerably well.

"If you are a philosopher you may become healthy, you may even attain to old age.

"If anything annoys you, ignore it; if anything is too much for you, have nothing to do with it; if others seek to drive you, go slowly and laugh at the fools who wish to worry you. What you can do comfortably, that do; what you cannot accomplish, do not bother yourself about, for our temporal circumstances are not improved by over-pressure of work. You only spend proportionately more on your domestic affairs, and so nothing is gained. Economy, limitation of superfluities (of which the hard worker has often very few) place us in a position to live with greater comfort—that is to say, more rationally, more intelligently, more in accordance with nature, more cheerfully, more quietly, more healthily. . . . Remain deaf to the bribery of praise, remain cold and pursue your own course slowly and quietly like a wise and sensible man. To enjoy with tranquil mind and body, that is what man is in the world for, and to do as much work as will procure him the means of enjoyment—certainly not to let himself be harassed and worn out with work. . . . You will see how healthy you will become by following my advice. . . . No horrible dreams disturb the sleep of him who lies down to rest with calm nerves, and the man who is free from care wakes in the morning without anxiety about the multifarious occupations of the day. What does he care? The happiness of life concerns him more than anything else. With fresh vigour he sets about his moderate work, and at his meals nothing, no ebullitions of blood, no cares, no solicitude of mind, hinders him from relishing what the beneficent Preserver of Life sets before him; and so one day follows another in quiet succession, until finally advanced age brings him to the termination of a well-spent life, and he rests serenely in another world as he has calmly lived in this one. . . . Farewell, follow my advice, and when all goes well with you, remember Dr. S. Hahnemann."

A postscript follows ending with the observation: "Conserved strength does not need to be renewed by medicine." This tailor of Gotha, in spite of a delicate constitution, lived to the age of ninety-two, and "Extracts" from Hahnemann's correspondence with him, which covered a number of years, were published in a small volume.

Perhaps one of the most valuable of this series of essays is an article *On Making the Body Hardy*. It sets an example not so much of moderation— a doubtful blessing in some connections—as of a sensitively swaying balance between alternatives which makes it a work we might well study to-day. The essay commences with some preliminary considerations of the degeneracy induced by luxury and a false refinement, including some Thackeray-like touches, as when he describes the farmer's daughter who, forsooth, cannot consider herself educated until she has acquired the blanched complexion of the French lady, and who "carries on an affected courtship with the downy-bearded young squire, Fritz, with his false calves, artificially enlarged thighs and coat padded with feathers; a striking contrast to the shirt of mail of his great-grandfather." Then follows a condemnation of those extremes with which those disgusted with such degeneracy seek to counteract it. He cites Hippocrates as having remarked on the fact that "changes from one extreme to another cannot be undertaken without danger" and therefore require great caution, observing that the hardening methods adopted by some bore a great resemblance to the incautious transference of hot-house plants in February. After this a passage tells us that "it is incredible what man can endure if he be gradually habituated to it." The Russian, the Negro, the Greenlander are then presented to us as enduring not only great extremes, but a swift transition from one to the other because they have from infancy been acclimatised to experiencing such.

"All these people," he observes shrewdly, "give their children no other education but their own example; they abandon them to their own will until they have attained a good age. It is much worse on the part of a teacher to err on the side of doing *too much* than *too little*. He may leave it to the free-will of the children to inure themselves; he does it before them, they imitate him, each according to his strength, and none must be forced to overstep the latter.

"The teacher cannot put himself in the situation of the boy, cannot enter thoroughly into his feelings, consequently the boy must be allowed to draw back when he wishes to do so. He will rather have sometimes to keep him back, for imitation is often too powerful a spur.

"It is best that these exercises should be carried on in the presence of the pupils only, without any spectator, for then all present will be animated by the same mind."

The same balancing of values is observed in Hahnemann's references to natural means of cure such as hydropathy. He writes: "If there exists anywhere a generally useful medicament, it is water." (The whole section relating to this matter in Supp. 38 of Haehl's Vol. II is of interest.)

Part of this small series of essays strictly belongs to a later time. One of its sections is a reprint of a letter to one of the ruling princes—"On the Choice of a Family Physician," whilst another on *Epidemics in General* anticipates our Town Planning movement:

"In towns about to be built houses higher than two stories should not be allowed, every street should be at least twenty paces in width and built quite straight, in order that the air may permeate it unimpeded, and behind every house there should be a courtyard and a garden as broad and twice as long as the house. In this way the air may be readily renovated, behind the houses in the considerable space formed by the adjoining gardens, and in front by the broad straight streets."

We may be sure that when laying down the measurements for the garden Hahnemann had only in view a legal minimum, which could become reasonably universal. There is an indication of his ability to make the most even of quite a little garden in an incident recorded during his subsequent residence in Köthen, where Dr. Lutze from Paris visited Hahnemann. The physician, it appears, allowed himself to comment on the smallness of the garden, of which he had heard a great deal previously, to which Hahnemann replied: "You are right. My garden is small. But, see how high it is!"

Dr. Haehl cites Pettenkofer, among his own countrymen, as having stated that "what was understood by hygiene in earlier times no longer applies" (here he mentions Hufeland, a contemporary of Hahnemann's). To this Haehl rightly adds that Pettenkofer should have made an exception of Hahnemann. His omission to name his remarkable teachings was no doubt attributable to ignorance of his works rather than to prejudice. This probably explains why Emil Kräpelin, also one of Hahnemann's countrymen, in his *One Hundred Years of Psychiatry* (1918), fails to cite him as a pioneer in the treatment of the mentally afflicted. History, indeed, not only requires to be written on all the available evidence, but the historian must ever be at work substantiating, revising, and supplementing his statements.

As dietist Hahnemann's philosophy is indicated by a "Dietetic Conversation," in which the partly serious, or if we will, partly witty observation occurs: "This article in our vital breviary is of such importance that it is certain that the beneficent Creator could not have founded it upon the shifting standard of the professional dietists; He must have given us infallible guiding principles to direct us in the selection of food and drink." This is not to say that Hahnemann despised a scientific enquiry into the question. "Grapes in the process of drying certainly lose important constituents which would be useful to the body," he writes in a note to Cullen's work, which also contains the observation: "The teaching of Pythagoras to limit the consumption of meat as much as possible has many points in its favour." But here as ever we shall find Hahnemann balancing generalities by a recognition of local conditions and custom as also by the recognition of individual idiosyncrasies and specific needs. An essay on *The Satisfaction of Our Animal Requirements* begins with the words "Man is manifestly made for enjoyment. . . . All creation around him is happy and rejoices; why should man, endowed with his finer sensibilities, not do so likewise?" Elsewhere Hahnemann observes that Hippocrates, because he wisely realised his imperfect knowledge of medicines, trusted largely to diet.

Yet whilst urging us to imitate Nature's method of producing "the greatest effect" with simple and often with small means, Hahnemann held that it was the privilege of man to use means unknown to Nature. In *The Medicine of Experience* he reminds us that the "great Instructor of Mankind suffers us not to employ the process of *sphacelus*, as the human corporeal organism does for itself, in order to remove a shattered limb, but he placed in our hand the sharp dividing knife which Faust moistened with oil, that is capable of performing the operation with less pain, less fever, and much less danger to life." These words were written after Hahnemann had discovered his new basis of medicine selection. This and other passages on the benefits of surgery, not alone for amputation but where necessary to meet various conditions, will dispose of the idea sometimes entertained that he was opposed to surgery.

How far Hahnemann believed in the *Vis Medicatrix Naturae*, the healing power of Nature within the human organism, has been a matter of controversy. This, because his remarks sometimes appear to be at variance with themselves. At one period he used the term "life force" only for the vital power by which the organism is maintained in health. Later he applied it also to the active life-principle asserting the patient's right to health in acute illnesses, whilst in chronic disease he saw all too clearly that the same vital powers of the patient have become more or less acquiescent. Yet even in such cases they could be awakened. "The powers of Nature," he wrote, "frequently accomplish wonderful, quick and beautiful cures. . . . Serious illnesses often get better of themselves . . . also in chronic affections this marvellous power of healing asserts itself." Far then from depreciating the healing powers of Nature, he sought nothing but the surest means of co-operating with them. With an imaginative ear, like that which enabled Michael Angelo to hear the voice of Beauty crying to be released in the rugged marble on the mountain side, this lover of humanity heard through the very symptoms of his patients the hidden life force, with its instinct for bodily vigour and beauty, giving "expression to its bondage and appealing for liberation to the understanding physician." But we are still at an era in Hahnemann's life when, to his sorrow, he could not reply to those appeals of the life force with any assurance of being able to render aid adequate to the need.

CHAPTER VII

THE NEW PRINCIPLE DECLARED

Königslutter, near Brunswick, 1796-1799

FROM Brunswick Hahnemann with his family now made his way to the comparatively small town of Königslutter near by, where he remained for about two and a half years. This period saw the publication of two significant essays, through the influence of which an "alternative" school of medicine was to emerge and establish itself throughout the old and the new world—a method of medicine selection which, from its inception, has only asked to be judged by its fruits. The first of these essays was entitled *On a New Principle for ascertaining the Curative Powers of Drugs*, the second *Are the Obstacles to Certainty and Simplicity in Practical Medicine Insurmountable?*

For six years Hahnemann had been testing his first intimations gained through the experiment with cinchona, and was now satisfied that he had lighted upon a perfectly reliable method of selecting medicines. But before this satisfaction was secured, with its promise of further attainments in the art of healing, Hahnemann passed through an extraordinary measure of mental suffering, due to his profound mistrust of the medical practices of his day. Many years later, in 1808, he recorded these in a powerful letter to his friend Hufeland, which we give here. It will be noticed that the eighteen years in retrospect, referred to in the opening passage, brings us back to the year of the cinchona experiment, *i.e.* to 1790.

"For eighteen years," he writes, "I have been deviating from the ordinary practice of medical art. My sense of duty would not easily allow me to treat the unknown pathological state of my suffering brethren with these unproved medicines. If they are not exactly suitable (and how could the physician know that, since they had not yet been proved?) they might, with their strong power, easily change life into death or induce new disorders and chronic maladies, often more difficult to eradicate than the original disease. The thought of becoming in this way a murderer or malefactor towards the life of my fellow human beings was most terrible to me, so terrible and disturbing that I gave up my practice in the first years of my married life. I scarcely treated anybody for fear of injuring him, and occupied myself solely with chemistry and writing.

"But then children were born to me, several children, and after a time serious illness occurred, which, in tormenting and endangering my children, my own flesh and blood, made it even more painful to my sense of duty, that I could not with any degree of assurance procure help for them. But whence was I to obtain help—certain and sure help—with our present knowledge of the power of medicines, resting as it does merely on vague observations, often merely on hypothetical opinions, and with the infinite number of arbitrary views of disease in our pathologies? This was a labyrinth, in which only that man can remain at ease who is willing to accept as truth the assertion of the healing powers of medicines, because they are printed in a hundred books, and who, without enquiry, receives as from an oracle the haphazard definitions of the diseases in the pathologies, as well as their cure in the hypothetical instances of our therapies. . . . 'Whence then was certain help to be obtained?' was the yearning cry of the comfortless father in the midst of the groaning of his children, dear to him above all else. Night and desolation around me—no sign of enlightenment for my troubled paternal heart.

"During my eight years' practice my attention had been repeatedly drawn to the delusion of the ordinary methods of healing, and I knew very well from sad experience what was to be hoped for from the methods of Sydenham and Hoffmann, from Boerhaave and Gaubius, or from Stoll, Quarin, Cullen and de Haen. Yet perhaps the whole nature of this science, as great men have already said, is such that it is not capable of any great certainty.

"What a shameful, blasphemous thought—I struck my brow—that the wisdom of the Infinite Spirit, animating the universe, should not be able to create means to pacify the sufferings of diseases which He, after all, allowed to arise!

"Would He, the Father of all, coldly survey the torments of disease in his dearest creatures? Would He leave open no way to the genius of mankind—otherwise so infallible—no easy, certain and dependable way of regarding disease from the right angle, of determining the use and the specific, safe and dependable results obtainable from medicines?

"Before I would have given credence to this blasphemy, I should have forsworn all the school systems of the world. . . .

"Well then, I thought, there must be a safe, more dependable method of healing, as sure as God is the wisest and most beneficent of beings; let me no longer seek it in the thorn hedges of existing statements, in arbitrary opinions and in false conclusions, even though they may adapt themselves wonderfully to a splendid system, nor yet in the authority of highly celebrated men full of delusions. No, let me seek it where it might be nearest at hand, and where they have all passed by, because it did not seem artificial or learned enough, and was not adorned with victorious laurel wreaths for its system, its pedantry or its far-fetched abstractions. It made its appeal only to me, who with no system nor any party to please, wished to be able to look on with normally easy conscience, should my endangered children die."

THE NEW PRINCIPLE DECLARED

Hahnemann has elsewhere also strong observations on the use of the term incurable except as a measure of human ignorance.

> "'Yes,' I hear the medical school whisper with a seemingly compassionate shrug, 'Yes, these are notoriously incurable evils; our books tell us they are incurable.' As if, indeed, it could comfort the millions of sufferers to be told of the impotence of our art! As if the Creator of these sufferers had not provided remedies for them also, and as if for them the source of boundless goodness did not exist, compared to which the tenderest mother's love is as thick clouds beside the glory of the noonday sun!"

Slowly then Hahnemann had arrived at the assurance that a demonstrable "law of cure" existed. The assumption that the existence of a "law of cure" would imply both a narrowness of concept and a hampering restriction in practice requires examination. To Hahnemann from the first the idea appeared in quite another light. For him, such a law would be capable of infinitely varied applications, as we shall see in following the lines of his research.

Judge Troward in *The Law and the Word* has expressed the matter admirably. He says:

> "When we first observe the working of the Law under conditions spontaneously provided by Nature, it appears to limit us; but by seeking the reason of the action exhibited under these conditions, we discover the principle and true

nature of the law in question, and we then learn from the law itself, what conditions to supply in order to give it more extended scope, and to direct its energy to the accomplishment of definite purposes. The maxim we have to learn is that 'Every law *contains in itself* the principle of its own expansion,' which will set us free from the limitation which that law at first appears to impose upon us. . . . The limitation was never in the law but in the conditions under which it was working, and our power of selection enables us to provide new conditions not provided by Nature and thus to *specialise* the law, and disclose immense powers which had always been latent in it, but which would forever remain hidden unless brought to light by the co-operation of the personal factor. The Law itself never changes, but we can specialise it by realising and providing the conditions thus indicated."

He instances the inviolable fact that iron cannot float in water, and proceeds to show us the ship that is built of iron floating because the shipbuilder has overcome the limitation which might appear to have been set, by making use of the law of displacement discovered by Archimedes. Similarly, in a world which, with all its new riches as regards knowledge of physics, still asserts the operation of Newton's "law of gravity" we see thistledown-lifted seeds floating, flames wrestling ever upwards and the blood of the venous system, in obedience to the other "law of pressure," upward bound.

In *Chemistry* we read that neither the Gay-Lussac law relating to the expansion of gases nor the law of Boyle relating to "pressure" in the same connection "is obeyed absolutely by all gases; there are departures depending primarily upon chemical idiosyncrasies." Whether such "departures" are actually departures from the given law or only "apparent departures" need not concern us here. It can be stated, however, that so insistent was Hahnemann on the importance of being aware of the likelihood of idiosyncrasies in the human organism, that despite his acceptance of a "law of cure," nothing whatever in the way of a foregone conclusion was to be entertained as regards response to treatment. He realised keenly the need of individualising. Even to get through to the reality which lies at the back of a patient's report Hahnemann appreciates the need of a fine penetration: "In all diseases and especially in chronic diseases, the discovery of the true and complete disease picture and of its individualities demands particular insight, scepticism, knowledge of human nature, wariness in enquiry, and patience of the profoundest kind."

With regard to the potentialities of drugs he observes: "Each substance effects alterations in the health and condition of the human body after its own distinct and definite fashion, a fashion which forbids the substitution of any other substance for itself."

In the first of the Essays referred to, that on the *Curative Power of Drugs*, Hahnemann writes:

"If I mistake not, practical medicine has devised three ways of applying remedies for the relief of disorders of the human body. The *first way, to remove or destroy the fundamental cause of the disease*, was the most elevated it could follow. All the imaginings and aspirations of the best physicians in all ages were directed to this object, the most worthy of the dignity of our art. But to use a Stagyrian expression, they did not advance beyond particulars; the great philosopher's stone, the knowledge of the fundamental cause of all diseases, they never attained to. . . ."

Despite the conspicuous importance given here and elsewhere by Hahnemann to the discovery and removal of the cause of ill-health, Allbutt in 1896 (*i.e.* since the appearance of Hahnemann's *Lesser Writings* in England) states: "He [Hahnemann] said that knowledge of pathology or of the causation of disease is useless."

Again the historian must have failed to consult original documents! Hahnemann, it is true, wrote in a note to the *Organon:* "All speculation and writing on the primary cause of disease is empty and remains idle boasting, it is a misleading play of the imagination." Such expressions may have been responsible for a misunderstanding in the mind of a casual student. But there remains the whole of his plea for the removal of bad social conditions and the recognition of germ life (which Hahnemann called *miasm*) as the cause of infections such as cholera, and his demands for isolation, etc.,

THE NEW PRINCIPLE DECLARED

together with pronouncements such as the above. No critical reader certainly should have been misled.

Hahnemann then proceeds:

"By the *second way*, the symptoms present were sought to be removed by medicines *which produced an opposite condition;* for example, constipation by purgatives; inflamed blood by venesection, cold and nitre; acidity in the stomach by alkalis; pains by opium. In acute diseases, which, if we remove the obstacles to recovery for but a few days, nature will herself generally conquer, or if we cannot do so, will succumb; in acute diseases, I repeat, this application of remedies is proper to the purpose and sufficient, as long as we do not possess the above-mentioned philosopher's stone (the knowledge of the fundamental cause of each disease, and the means of its removal), or as long as we have no rapidly acting specific, which would extinguish the variolous infection at its very commencement. In this case, I would call such remedies *temporary*.

"But should the fundamental cause of the disease, and its direct means of removal, be known to us, and we, disregarding these, combat the symptoms only by remedies of this second kind, or employ them seriously in chronic diseases, then this method of treatment (to combat diseases by remedies that produce an opposite state) gets the name of palliative, and is to be rejected. In chronic diseases it only gives relief at first; subsequently stronger doses become necessary, which cannot remove the primary disease, and thus they do more harm the longer they are employed, for reasons to be specified hereafter."

The fact that Hahnemann adopted the word "palliative" to signify the mistaken use of the law of contraries in medicine selection has led some to suppose that he was against the swift alleviation of suffering, in other words that he was, under all circumstances, against palliating pain by the use of drugs. The above shows conclusively that this was not so. As a purely temporary measure he sanctioned it, but he preferred to call this use of contraries (such as opium for the relief of pain) *temporary*, lest palliative methods should be regarded, as they customarily were, as the sole requirement in any treatment.

Hahnemann then proceeds in his essay to describe the method of his own choice, namely: "*that in order to discover the true remedial powers of a medicine, we must look to the specific artificial disease it can develop in the [healthy] human body, and employ it in a similar morbid condition of the organism which it is wished to remove.*" He then continues to remind his readers that in his additions to Cullen's *Materia Medica*, he had already observed that cinchona bark, given in large doses to sensitive yet healthy individuals, produces a true attack of fever, very similar to the intermittent fever, and for this reason probably it overpowers and thus cures the latter, adding: "Now after mature experience, I add, not only *probably* but *quite certainly*." This certainty was derived from the close comparison of disease symptoms produced by a variety of drugs tested first upon himself and afterwards on other healthy persons, and the beneficial effects of the same drugs used in cases of sickness which showed similar symptoms. When Hahnemann says elsewhere "the more similar the better," he is referring to the resemblance between the totality of the various symptoms the drug can produce on the healthy and the totality of those symptoms in the disease which it is desired to cure.

In the course of ordinary practice Hahnemann was accustomed to the fact that "most medicines have more than one action; the first a *direct* action, which generally changes into the second." This he called "the indirect, secondary action." In a note to the passage referring to this in the essay Hahnemann instances opium. This drug he shows us at first producing "a fearless elevation of spirit, a sensation of strength and high courage, an imaginative gaiety," but after some hours have passed we find the person so elevated as a first result of taking the drug "relaxed, dejected, peevish, with confused memory and generally discomforted and fearful." The last state of that man is then certainly "worse than the first."

Hahnemann therefore welcomed, as a first action, some accentuation of the patient's symptoms, because experience had taught him that where this was the nature of the direct action, the secondary or indirect action decided in favour of a reduction in the symptoms and in cure. This initial aggravation where, consciously or unconsciously, homœopathic remedies have been used, is now often identified with Wright's "negative phase." This was the name given by Sir Almroth Wright to the aggravation that may follow a dose of a vaccine.

But not only did Hahnemann anticipate later scientific discovery in this matter. As was his wont he himself hastened to tell us that he had been anticipated. A note to the above section states: "This aggravation, an exaltation of the drug symptoms over the analogous disease symptoms, has been observed by other physicians when by chance they have employed a homœopathic remedy."

The method of prescribing according to the law of similars Hahnemann had named "homœopathy" from the Greek words *homoion*—similar, and *pathos*—disease. All treatment by the then universally accepted "law of contraries" he termed "allopathy," from *alloion*, meaning "of a different kind" or contrary. Where the two terms appear from now they must be understood to indicate respectively these two methods of medicine selection. Every follower of Hahnemann uses the first as the basis of his practice, and treats by contraries only as a rare and temporary expedient.

The "nine points" of Hufeland, Hahnemann's most distinguished contemporary, in favour of homœopathy may be cited here, though, as none of them actually refer to the "law of similars" itself, we need not regard them as more than enumerations of important attendant advantages. They were:

"I. It will attract attention to the all-important question of individualisation.

II. It will help to bring dietetics back to its own.

III. It will prohibit large doses of medicine.

IV. It will lead to simplification of prescriptions.

V. It will lead to more accurate testing and determination of the effect of remedies on the living subject, as it has to a certain extent already done.

VI. The homœopathic process will direct attention more to the preparations and bring about a stricter supervision of the apothecaries.

VII. It will never do positive injury.

VIII. It will give the sick organism more time for quiet and undisturbed self-help.

IX. It will lessen the cost of curing to an extraordinary extent."

Hufeland also expressed what were to him definite objections to the new method, the most important of which was perhaps the first: "The homœopathic process of healing may lead to a merely symptomatic (purely empiric) type of cure, and may suppress the causal method, which is the basis of all rational medical practice."

To anyone who had read Hahnemann's declaration that in medicine there were no specifics for diseases, but as many specifics as there were symptoms of disease, such an apprehension was not unnatural. Yet Hufeland was wise enough to couch this criticism in the phrase of a problematic prophecy—"may lead to"—

and for us the answer can only be found in an examination of the homœopathic hospitals throughout the world where each and every device for exact diagnosis and surgical and other treatments are to be found in association with Hahnemann's precise method of medicine selection according to the law *similia similibus curentur*.

Hufeland's observations for and against homœopathy end with the beautiful reflection: "Time will judge. Till then we will continue to test without prejudice, keep more to the facts than to theory and above all found no new sects, endowed with intolerance and a desire to persecute! Let us all consider ourselves as acolytes of one temple, who are striving after one common aim, even though it may be along different paths."

In the realm of the natural sciences as well as of medicine itself, we find that Hahnemann's range of interest was at once intensive and wide. Records of previous centuries and of all lands, held, as we have seen, his interest and called forth his powers as an original commentator as well as translator. We find in Hahnemann also a keen critic as to the "authenticity" of ancient writings. He held more than one of the works then still attributed to Hippocrates to be either spurious or misnamed. (*Vide* Notes to the Edinburgh Review article entitled *Hahnemann's Homœopathy*, Jan. 1830.) Chemistry was of profound interest, and in the work entitled the *Curative Powers of Drugs* his appreciation of botany as a field of research for the physician reappears. One part of the essay is a review of the opposite effects which may be derived from plants belonging botanically to one family.

"In the family of *coniferae*, the inner bark of the fir tree (*pinus sylvestris*) gives to the inhabitants of the Northern regions a kind of bread, whereas the bark of the yew tree (*taxus baccifera*) gives—death. ... And again, in the family *solanaceae*, how comes the tasteless great mullein (*verbascum thapsus*) along with the burning Cayenne pepper (*capsicum annuum*)?"

The healing virtues of herbs has a fascination which might well detain us, a subject which has not escaped even the mind of the poets. Thus Meredith, for instance, in *Phoebus with Admetus*, writes of: "Tales of search for simples and those who sought of love," and later exclaims:

"Lo! the herb of healing, when once the herb is known,
  Shines in shady woods bright as new-sprung flame"

whilst his poem *Melampus*—physician and sage—is filled with a sense of Nature's healing gift, in its wider working, through the

"Glory of vision, honey, the breeze
  In heat, the run of the river on root and stone."

In Hahnemann's later dissertation before the Leipzig professors on the *Helleborism of the Ancients*, we find that the most famous cure ascribed to Melampus was achieved by an application of the law of similars. This, as the old historians narrate it, was as follows:

"About the year 1500 before our era a certain Melampus, son of Amithaon, a most celebrated augur and physician, first at Pylos, then among the Argives, is said to have cured the daughters of Proteus, King of the Argives, who in consequence of remaining unmarried were seized with an amorous furor and affected by a wandering mania; they were cured chiefly by means of veratrum album, given in the milk of goats fed upon veratrum. . . . From this circumstance the great fame of this plant is derived."

As this plant (the hellebore) could also cause mania, the story was of two-fold interest to Hahnemann.

Far from desiring to lay claim to any superficial originality even as regards the basic principle of his method, Hahnemann made it part of his task to unearth from the writings of others instances in which, recognised or unrecognised, the law of similars had operated in medicine throughout the past. He drew attention to the fact that he had been anticipated by a number of physicians throughout the ages, notably by the Hippocratic writings, as in *Places in Man*. Of this work, Dr. W. H. S. Jones, editor of the new *Loeb* edition of the works of Hippocrates, says: "*Places in Man* is apparently of the fourth century B.C. . . . while not belonging to the great group of (apparently) genuine works, it is not unlike other 'almost' Hippocratic treatises in its medical doctrines." He adds that chapters XL-XLVI are "interesting chapters on the philosophy of medicine, including some account of *homœopathy*." It was pointed out to

Hahnemann later that this was true also of Paracelsus.

Garrison, in his *History of Medicine*, published in 1929, unfortunately states that Hahnemann, "as the result of certain experiments . . . began to formulate those theories which characterise his system. These are, first, a revival of the old Paracelsian doctrine of 'signature,' namely, that diseases or symptoms of disease are curable by those particular drugs which produce similar pathological effects upon the body. . . ." We instance this confusion of the "doctrine of signature" with "the law of similars"—two totally different things—because it may have accounted for the supposition that Hahnemann utilised the doctrine of signature in his selection of medicines. The author of *Devils, Drugs and Doctors*, indeed, quite definitely states this. He says: "In selecting some of his drugs he [Hahnemann] employed the principle of so-called 'signatures,' which he borrowed from Paracelsus. This theory is based on the astrological conception that the stars impress the 'signature' of disease upon drugs. It was believed that this 'signature' can be recognised from the form and colour of the plant from which the drug is obtained." He then names one or two cases where such likeness exists, as in the flower eye-bright from which *Euphrasia*, an eye remedy, is actually distilled.

This is not the place to discuss the various remarkable coincidences in medicines which led to this doctrine. We must, however, show that as a principle upon which to rely in medicine selection, Hahnemann definitely rejected it. In his *Materia Medica Pura* we read under *Chelidonium* (celandine): "The ancients imagined that the yellow colour of the juice of this plant was an indication (signature) of its utility in bilious diseases. The moderns from this extended its employment to hepatic diseases. . . . The importance of human health does not admit of any such uncertain directions for the employment of medicines. It would be criminal frivolity to rest contented with such guesswork at the bedside of the sick. Only that which the drugs themselves unequivocally reveal of their peculiar powers in their effects on the healthy—that is to say, only their pure symptoms—can teach us loudly and clearly when they can be advantageously used with certainty. . . ."

Because the principle of similars which he advocated for general adoption had been brought into play previously by others, Hahnemann has been regarded by some as a mere plagiarist posing as an original thinker. The best answer to this accusation comes to us from the pen of Dr. August Bier, Privy Counsellor and Professor of Medicine in the Berlin University. He says, "Even Hahnemann's priority in homœopathy has been questioned in a preposterous manner. . . This is totally out of the question. Neither the teachings of Hippocrates nor of Paracelsus have exerted an influence towards the practical application of the law of similars, its sole founder being Hahnemann."

CHAPTER VIII

THE HIPPOCRATES OF THE INFINITELY LITTLE

Years covered by Chapters VII and IX

To Hahnemann the values of his world were clearly becoming less and less determined by weight and size, more and more dependent on those fine adjustments in measure which are essential to the harmonious working of the various factors which influence the whole of life in its three interrelated spheres of body, mind and spirit. With Blake-like simplicity and penetration he wrote of "the fatherly goodness of Him for whom no sufficiently worthy name can be found, who tends all and cares for the infinitesimal needs of the little animals in the dust, invisible to the sharpest human eye. . . ."

There is evidence that by the time these reflections were penned Hahnemann knew the writings of the eminent physician Boerhaave. This writer was responsible for the publication of the entomological writings of Swammerdam who, because of his contributions to the actual adaptations of the microscope and his microscopical research, has been called "the Galileo of the Infinitely Little." It is likely, therefore, that Hahnemann may have been familiar with and influenced by the work of the great Dutch naturalist.

The discovery of a heightened power to cure with an increasing smallness of dose affected Hahnemann profoundly. It became for him something approaching a revelation of the Creative Mind. Poisons, he found, could be reduced to such an extent as not only to be completely redeemed from their noxious character, but so as to be endowed with curative virtues far excelling in some instances those of the more obviously benevolent substances. He saw that it was to our clumsy use of them alone that they owed their ill-repute. "The Creator of infinitely manifold nature is not on this account to be blamed if, for example, saltpetre is so constituted that it is not possible to swallow handfuls without danger to life." This was written, perhaps, not without a touch of quiet humour.

"Has He," Hahnemann asks, "perchance established a law that we should regard the scruple, the grain, as the smallest and most suitable dose of all medicines? Has He not rather delivered into our hands means of obtaining smaller and ever smaller doses of the more potent and most potent substances? ... Who will prevent us from doing this and so adapting our needs wisely to the potency of the different drugs? The fact that medicines only become suitable curative media for the human body, when administered in different quantities, is to the wise man no reason why the more potent drugs, useful only in smaller doses, should straightway be dismissed as poison. . . . Where the public sees only objects of abhorrence, the wise man beholds objects worthy of the deepest veneration and avails himself of them, whilst adoring the Eternal Source of Love. Sapere aude."

We need not mistrust these expressions as those of some impracticable visionary. The same pen that inscribed them wrote also, it must be remembered, the work on *Arsenic and its Forensic Detection*, laying down precise restrictions for the sale of that poison. No one appreciated better than Hahnemann the need of warning against misuse of such substances, sublime though he acknowledged their uses to be if used in appropriate measure. "He is to learn a divine art that would now be happy," wrote Thomas Traherne in another connection, "and that is, like a royal chemist to reign among poisons." How expressive are these words of what was to become increasingly the experience of this Saxon physician, who might well be called the "Hippocrates of the Infinitely Little."

In other realms than medicine Hahnemann recognised that identical substances may be used for ill or good. Inspired by contemplation of this fact, he wrote:

"When the All-blessed created iron, he accorded the children of men ability to make from it either the murderous dagger or the gentle ploughshare, and therewith to slay or to nourish their brethren. How much happier they would make themselves by applying His gifts only for beneficence's sake! This was the purpose of their lives, this was His will."

All records of overdosing at this period became of absorbing interest to Hahnemann, and we can imagine with what interest he would have studied the work of the Berlin Professor Lewin.

One of the most noted instances of a medicine selected and publicly recommended by Hahnemann to his colleagues on the ground of its being a "similar" was belladonna for scarlet fever. This medicine, moreover, he administered in a very high potency, that is in an infinitesimal dose.

Hahnemann tells us how he first lighted upon the remedial virtues of belladonna in the course of his practice. At a time of epidemic a mother had unwittingly bought a new counterpane from a seamstress, who, without declaring the fact, had a child sick with scarlet fever in her room. The house into which the infected counterpane was brought contained a large family of children, and a daughter fell ill several days after, presenting a wide number of symptoms. Hahnemann was called in to the case.

"My memory, and my written collection of the peculiar effects of some medicines," he wrote, "furnished me with no remedy so capable of producing a counterpart of the symptoms here present as belladonna. . . . I therefore gave this girl of ten years of age, who was already affected by the first stages of scarlet fever, a dose of this medicine (1/432,999th part of a grain of the extract, which, according to my subsequent experience, is rather too large a dose). So remarkable was the effect that the following day she was playing again, complaining of nothing and quite lively, though meanwhile two of the other children had sickened without my knowledge."

This case, to which only a few further doses at some intervals were prescribed, led him to reason that what could arrest an illness at an early stage might also be the best preventive. The doctor then recollected that some weeks previously he had visited a family where three children lay stricken with scarlet fever, the eldest daughter alone, who had been taking belladonna on account of quite a different affection, not having sickened. And this although during previous epidemics the eldest daughter had shown a disposition to take them first. He straightway, therefore, gave to the remaining five children of the family he was now attending very small doses of the drug every seventy-two hours, and they all remained well throughout the epidemic, in spite of the presence of their badly infected sisters in the house, for their removal had been impossible. After this, a number of other opportunities presented themselves to him, where this specific preventive remedy never failed.

The publicity which Hahnemann gave to this "providential discovery" led to very severe attacks. These were, it is true, directed mainly to the smallness of the dose. It was even stated publicly that his powders contained no belladonna at all. Some physicians went so far as to apply his remedy to a different type of fever, announcing, for all the world to hear, that Hahnemann's prescription had failed!

The attacks were so violent that even his most faithful of friends, Councillor Becker of Gotha, did not know what to make of him. This time the business interests and the good name of Becker were also attacked, because of the publication of Hahnemann's articles in his "Reichsanzeiger." For that reason Hahnemann went into the different points of the accusation in two letters at length. . . . The explanations offered seem to have been effective upon his friend, for in the year 1801 his work *Cure and Prevention of Scarlet Fever* was published by Becker.

The unfair way in which the accusations were fought out in public was complained of by Hahnemann in the same year in his essay *View of Professional Liberality at the Commencement of the Nineteenth Century*. This included an appeal equal in generosity of feeling to that of Hufeland for a united quest for truth, ending with the words "Physicians of Germany, be brothers, be fair, be just."

Even as far on as the year 1821 the doctor had to defend himself once more in this matter. But in various quarters, as time went on, the value of belladonna in scarlet fever received more recognition from the medical profession. In 1825 Hufeland published a work entitled *The Prophylactic Effect of Belladonna*, ascribing the discovery of this efficacious remedy for scarlet

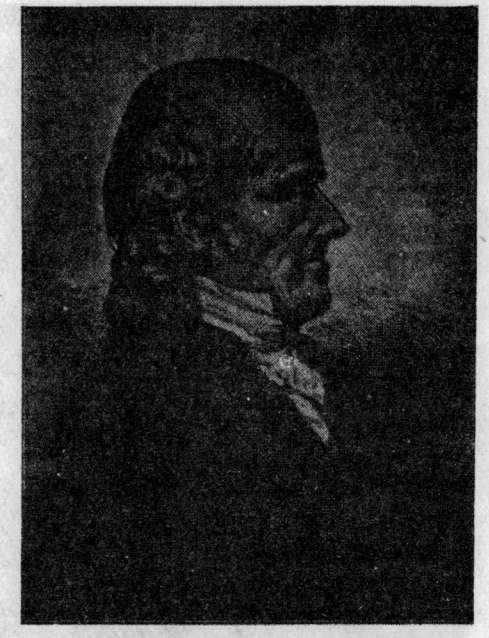

HAHNEMANN, FROM AN ETCHING
(*Probably the copper-plate referred to in his letter to Bönninghausen*)
(*See page 265*)

Faces pages 144

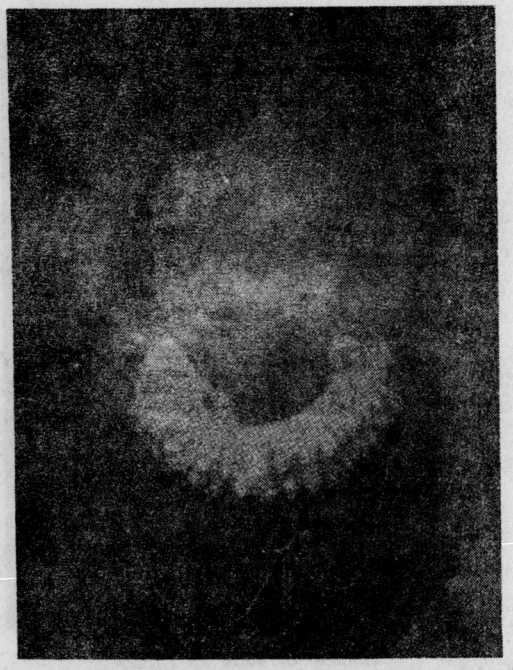

HAHNEMANN'S DAUGHTER CHARLOTTE: ONE OF THE TWO WHO LIVED LONGEST WITH HIM.

See page 261 *Faces page 145*

fever to Hahnemann. Thirteen years later the Prussian Government ordered the doctors of the country to use belladonna in small doses against the epidemics of scarlet fever which were very prevalent at that time.

As clinical experience proved that the medicinal virtues were undoubtedly increased by the processes of attenuation, trituration and succussion, Hahnemann called those processes *potentisation*, that is, a making more potent for cure though less powerful for harm.

The law which he was thus utilising had not been defined up to that time. It is now known as the Arndt-Schulz law. In *The Case for Homœopathy* it is thus formulated: "To any given stimulus, thermal, electrical, chemical (*e.g.* drug administration) protoplasm reacts differently according to the dosage of the stimulus. Small doses encourage life activity; large doses impede life activity; very large doses destroy life activity." Hahnemann was now further assured that the greater the power of the medicinal substance to cause harm in large quantities, the greater also its potentiality for good if given in sufficiently small measure and prepared by the necessary method. It is impossible to treat of this at any length here, but it will be sufficient to say that to it Hahnemann looked for the dynamization of all substances used. For Hahnemann in no sense, as some have supposed, confined his researches to the vegetable kingdom. Metallurgy had interested him from the Hettstedt days, and it was "by grinding down insoluble substances until they could be used as remedial agents, and reducing his 'like' medicines till aggravation in the patient's symptoms became negligible, that Hahnemann stumbled upon potentisation." "Thus," he wrote, "pure gold, silver, platina, have no action on the health in their solid state—nor crude vegetable charcoal, etc. . . . These substances are in a state of suspended animation as regards the medicinal action. But triturate one grain of gold leaf with 100 grains of sugar of milk, and a preparation results which has already great medicinal power." In addition to vegetable and mineral preparations Hahnemann also used disease poisons in infinitesimal dosage. After undergoing his processes these became, he held, "just as much altered as gold," and from Hahnemann's day on homœopaths have been using them for the cure of disease.

Hahnemann was eager that this alteration, resulting from "potentisation," should be recognised, lest his law of "similars" should be confused with treatment by "identicals." The possibility of this confusion was increased by an erroneous rendering sometimes used for the name of his principle in medicine selection. "What an immense amount of learning," he wrote, "do not my critics display! I shall only allude to those who write and print 'homopathic' and 'homopathy,' in place of homœopathic and homœopathy, thereby betraying that they are not aware of the immense difference between ὁμὸν (homon) and ὅμοιον (homoion), but consider the two to be synonymous. Did they never hear a word about, what the whole world knows, how the infinite difference between ὁμοούσιος (homoousios) and ὁμοιούσιος (homoiousios) once split the whole Christian Church into two parts, impossible to be re-united? Do they not understand enough Greek to know that (alone and in combination) ὁμὸν means common, identical, the same (e.g. εἰς ὁμὸν λέχος εἰσαναβαίνοι—*Iliad*), but that ὅμοιον only means similar, resembling the object, but *never* becoming identical with it? The homœopathic doctrine never pretended to cure a disease by the *same*, the *identical* power by which the disease was produced."

In the year 1797 Hahnemann was already able to state that for several years he had never prescribed more than one medicine at a time. He adds: "And I have never repeated a dose until the effect of the previous one had been exhausted." His reason for thus acting was, to use his own words, that "the human mind never understands more than one thing at a time . . ." By drug isolation he sought to "learn exactly in every case what the medicine has achieved, so that it could be used again in similar cases with the same or even greater success." These extracts we take from *Are the Obstacles to Certainty and Simplicity Insurmountable?* in which essay he further questions:

"Is it really more learned to prescribe from the chemist's shop a number of complicated combinations of medicines for one disease (often in one day) . . . ? Methinks to give the right remedy, not the many mixed, were the stroke of art. Hippocrates sought the simplest from out an entire genus of diseases; this he carefully observed and accurately described. In these simplest diseases he gave simple remedies from the scanty store then available. Thus he was enabled to see what he saw—to do what he did. I hope it will not be considered unfashionable to go to work with diseases as simply as did this truly great man."

Each new feature in Hahnemann's contribution to medicine—and there were yet others to come—increased the opposition. To prescribe only one medicine at a time in his day was unthought of. Every prescription had to consist of a basis (*constituens*), a supporting part (*adjuvans*) and a taste-improving part (*corrigens*). In a single prescription ten, twenty, thirty, or even a greater number of medicines were sometimes mixed together, whilst doctors who did not wish to exercise their own selective faculties could buy the so-called "magistral formulas" composed by physicians of note, and kept in store by the apothecaries. All medicines were administered frequently and in large doses, and changed every two or three days, or in acute cases every day.

"The ordinary observer," Hahnemann wrote in later years, "has no conception how extraordinarily sensitive the body becomes to drugs when it is diseased and especially to drugs chosen homœopathically. . . . The action upon the living human body of the remedial counter-force, which constitutes a medicine, is so profound and spreads from those sensitive areas well supplied with nerves, to which it is first applied, throughout the whole organism with such inconceivable rapidity and completeness that this action must be called spiritlike! It is almost as spiritlike as the action of vitality itself, by which its power is reflected on the organism."

The great variety and quantity of drugs that entered the already disordered system was not unnaturally a matter of dismay to a man of Hahnemann's penetration and concern for the sick. No wonder that he was led to exclaim, "O! that I might succeed in directing the better kind of doctor—him who sympathises with the suffering of our brethren and longs to be able to help them—to purer principles leading directly to the goal."

In Singer's *Short History of Medicine* we read: "Polypharmacy, the giving of many drugs together, is a vice from which medicine has now in large part freed itself." In Hahnemann standing thus alone in Germany and, indeed, in Europe towards the close of the eighteenth century, we cannot fail to recognise a pioneer of the reform by means of which medicine in large part set itself free. As is usual, the progress towards better things had to be set in motion by strenuous individual labours and a willingness to gather into one breast all the spearheads of opposition, as did the famous legendary warrior of old.

Hahnemann's handling of the subject of his

medicinal substances closely resembled the manner in which Cennino Cennini, an Italian painter, somewhat later than Giotto, regarded the materials of his art. Cennino has left us his directions for the preparation of vegetable and mineral substances for use in the painting of pictures, explaining how by various degrees of pulverisation their peculiar beauties could be released. Of the blue made from grinding lapis lazuli to a powder Cennino speaks as "noble, beautiful, and perfect beyond all other colours," whilst Hahnemann writes in the same vein of the "noble simplicity of pure gold." The fact that in some cases their substances, such as cinnabar and gold, were the same carries the analogy further.

On the question of the healing properties of gold Hahnemann wrote: "Modern physicians have pronounced this to be inactive; they have at length expunged it from all their Materia Medicas, and thereby deprived us of its mighty curative virtues." "At first," he continues, "I allowed myself to be deterred by these deniers from hoping for medicinal properties in pure gold." He then embarked on experiments with gold, and parallel with practical work his literary researches continued. "I was delighted to find," he writes, "a number of Arabian physicians unanimously testifying to the medicinal powers of gold in a finely pulverised form, particularly in some serious morbid conditions, in some of which the solution of gold had already been of great use to me." Later he states that: "even small doses of this metal given in the form mentioned caused in healthy adults morbid states very similar to those cured." He therefore deduced that these Orientals who had recorded its serviceableness in such disorders had been acting in an "unconscious homœopathic manner."

On this question Hahnemann closes with the exclamation: "Poor, fabulous Materia Medica of the ordinary stamp, how far dost thou lag behind the revelation which medicines in their action on the healthy human body clearly make!"

In his instructions for the grinding of gold for medicinal purposes finely enough to pass into something approaching a soluble state, this Saxon doctor, it is now recognised, anticipated the making of "colloids." Hahnemann's solitary and valuable experiments were, however, met by most of his colleagues with indifference or scorn.

"We must remember," says Dr. Neish Barker in *Hahnemann the Pioneer*, "that their knowledge was scant and their instruments imperfect. We may even sympathise with them in their opposition to the revolutionary doctrines of Hahnemann. Are we so open-minded and far-seeing as readily to scrap our cherished beliefs, even if a prophet were to rise among us?"

Hahnemann, like all other men who have been in advance of their age, had opponents of very varied dispositions, both the sincere and the insincere.

Yet however hard it may have been for his

contemporaries, we are to-day at a greater advantage in our capacity to appreciate scientifically his intuitive reckoning with the significance of the minute. In the chapter on "Atomic Weights" in Raphael Meldola's *Chemistry*, we read that "there has been added to the resources of the physicist and chemist a micro-balance constructed of quartz capable of weighing the almost inconceivably small quantity of 1-250,000th of a milligram." Hahnemann had no such laboratory apparatus, but by reckoning with the reality of the infinitesimal he had the joy of seeing patients recover from diseases which he had not previously been able to cure.

The demonstrable power of imperceptible quantities in some cases to cause harmful effects, will be familiar to all who have had modern industrial experience. An article which appeared in the *British Medical Journal* of June 1st, 1929, entitled "Amblyopia in the Artificial Silk Factory" stated:

> "It is disquieting to hear of a case of amblyopia contracted in an artificial silk factory, and to read, in a recent report of the Chief Inspector of Factories, of a case involving 'headache, vomiting, delirium, loss of muscular power and almost complete loss of sensation.' The trouble occurs in what is called the 'churn' room, where the alkali-cellulose is treated with carbon bisulphide in a hermetically sealed mixer or churn. . . . Few workers in the churn room are free from slighter symptoms, attributable to carbon bisulphide;

nor is this surprising, *seeing that 0.3 per 10,000 of air* will produce them."

Obviously a substance so powerful for harm in such small quantities as the above would require great attenuation to become potent for good according to the Arndt-Schultz law. That law, as we have shown, Hahnemann lighted upon and was wise enough to prize in practice before Rudolf Arndt formulated the rule as a biologist and Hugo Schultz adopted it as the basis of his therapeutics.

As an indication of the degree in which Hahnemann anticipated modern science, we may close this chapter with an extract from *The Practitioner* for October, 1928:

"Physical sciences teach that there are great forces (potencies) which are entirely imponderable like light and heat. . . . Were Hahnemann alive in this age, to which he belongs, he would find confirmation in the pathological and therapeutic effects of X-rays and radium—'imponderables' and, by their antagonistically malign and benign actions, perfectly exemplifying his law. The chemistry of our day is more and more approaching Hahnemann, with its colloids and ions, its ferments and vitamins. The infinitely little is becoming the infinitely potent, and bulk and energy of particle are seen to be in inverse ratio."

CHAPTER IX

"ÆSCULAPIUS IN THE BALANCE"

Hamburg-Altona, Mölln, Machern, Eilenburg, Dessau, Torgau

1799-1811

HAHNEMANN's nomadic character was to be still further shown by a succession of migrations. From Königslutter, where he stayed till 1799, he went to Hamburg-Altona. Here he made a fresh attempt to cure the mentally afflicted by receiving into his home the Viennese dramatist, Johann Karl Wezel, who was in favour with Kaiser Joseph II, and in whose welfare a circle of literary friends were especially concerned. The disposition of this patient, however, proved to be the opposite of the reports given to Hahnemann, and it became evident that his case was unsuited to treatment in a private house. Immediately following this episode a year was spent in Mölln, near Lauenburg. On his arrival there, Hahnemann says:

> "Hamburg would ruin any honest man who was not in commerce. Thank goodness, I came here, where I need earn only half the amount in order to live with more comfort than in Hamburg. It is a small place with

230 houses, mostly filled with modest working people, and possessing all necessary requirements amid beautiful surroundings. Here I will again stand at the helm of the little ship of my making, and only cure what Heaven sends me. The huge merciless waves of Hamburg which carry huge vessels but overturn small craft had almost swallowed me up."

The letter then reverts to the subject of his recently dismissed patient:

"If I did not directly help the unhappy man, who is very different from what has been said about him, I may be able to help him indirectly, leaving it to you and circumstances to decide. I know him sufficiently now to be able to give good advice more easily than others could do, and will do so free of charge."

The exclamation follows: "Oh! if only we had escaped the war, which is the grave of science."

From Mölln Hahnemann with his wife and children then roamed to Machern and Eilenburg, near Leipzig, retiring from there to Dessau, where he had met Henrietta Küchler, who during the intervening years had proved so invaluable a wife. Some have ascribed to this strong-charactered housewife an almost tyrannical nature. Yet Samuel Hahnemann expected her to hold the reins of government in her own hands so far as household matters went. Indeed, one so preoccupied as he could hardly have done otherwise. To detect that her life was not an easy one demands little imaginative faculty. Haehl writes:

"Deprivation of every sort, even oppressive need and hunger dominated for a long time the family of the young doctor and scholar, whose wife had come from more opulent circumstances as an apothecary's daughter. But the roots of her being spread into the hard ground in which she was planted, and her strong, energetic will overcame all difficulties."

That the Hahnemann family had now entered a more prosperous period is shown by the fact that in Machern we find the doctor occupying a house of his own. A description of poverty given by one of the Hahnemann relatives to Dr. Dudgeon as belonging to this time should undoubtedly have referred to an earlier era. As it is common for prosperity to follow, rather than precede days of hardship, unfortunately even these more prosperous times usually inherit some legacy of strain.

Yet in various ways it is clear that the relationship between Hahnemann and his wife remained throughout rich in understanding. In the earlier years of their marriage Samuel Hahnemann had been able to write: "Four daughters and one son, together with my wife, form the spice of my life." And throughout we find expressions of the same happy conception of the married state alike from the standpoint of the husband and the wife. To a medical colleague on the occasion of his marriage he wrote: "Both perfect each other, and love, mutual help, warning and advice help us to bear the burden of life easily and procure for us a condition as nearly akin to paradise as is possible on earth."

Perhaps no more penetrating glance into the domestic sphere and the spirit in which Hahnemann interpreted its events can be found than in a long letter written later to a disciple, Dr. Stapf, on the anticipation of the birth of another child. After referring to the perils of childbirth, he continues:

"Behold! what great and solemn preparations for the arrival of its new citizen into this world. . . .—a young life of divine origin. I, at least, have been deeply touched in my innermost soul by each of these almost superphysical events, . . . and have accepted it as a process of moral purification from the great Principle of Goodness, the Father of all perfected souls, and have endeavoured to utilise these awe-inspiring moments, obviously meant for eternity, for the cleansing and purification of my character. And where there was yet left a blemish of jealousy for my fellow-brethren, or a fold in my heart which concealed a suspicion of deceit, or any trace of untruth and falsehood, or where I detected a tendency to appear different or to talk otherwise than coincided with my inner conviction, I have swept it away. In these hours I have always vowed to cultivate simplicity, honesty and truth, and to find contentment and happiness in the eyes of the Great Father of all life, on the one hand, by ever perfecting the innermost growth of the soul, as is seemly for a citizen of eternity, and on the other hand, by making those around me happy. . . ."

To Councillor Becker during these years of migration from one township to another he wrote:

> "They could just as well blame me for the frequent changes of my residence, as they could any other traveller: 'Why not remain on the same spot like the coral polyp?' To the external circumstances of a scholar, only a man of feeble intellect would take exception; whether a man wear a round wig or a plait instead of the usual 'Swedish' head, whether he wear boots or shoes, what has it to do with them? The unbiassed man remembers the story of the goldsmith's boy, and laughs. The greatest criminals might deserve to remain chained to their birthplace! To whom do I owe anything if I go away elsewhere? Let him come forward whom I have cheated out of a penny. Who gives me the money for the journey (the last one cost 7,000 thalers) that he should have the right to ask where I am going?"

Haehl is no doubt right when he ascribes the nomadic habit in Hahnemann to a variety of causes, though he sweeps aside altogether one possible contributory factor, perhaps a little too finally. He says:

> "The suggestion that the artistic temperament, so marked in his own family, had possibly developed in him the restless inclination for travelling, cannot be taken into serious consideration, if we recall the fact that the grandfather, father and uncle were

rooted in the towns in which they dwelt quite as firmly as artizans."

But surely it is after all just here that the difference lay. His father and uncle at least were induced by circumstances to remain in one locality. There was no such fetter on Samuel Hahnemann. On the contrary, there was everything to drive him forth from one neighbourhood to another. In one place he could not earn sufficient, in another he was beset with unfriendly critics, in another the price of food and other essentials was exorbitant. Add an artistic temperament to these and his other incentives to wander, and who shall say that this inherited disposition may not have been largely responsible for his yielding so readily to each successive spur.

In spite of wide recognition as a chemist Hahnemann at about this time, 1800-1, made, and made publicly, one serious mistake in chemistry. This was seized upon by his opponents and utilised to injure his reputation. Even as late as 1853 Dr. James Young Simpson, of Edinburgh, famous as the first to apply chloroform as an anæsthetic, unacquainted with anything but a garbled version of this incident in Hahnemann's life, unfortunately turned the suspicion cast by his contemporaries into the crystallised mis-statement: "We know at least that Hahnemann once deceived people."

Believing he had found by certain combinations a new alkaline salt, Hahnemann had announced the supposed discovery in no fewer than three

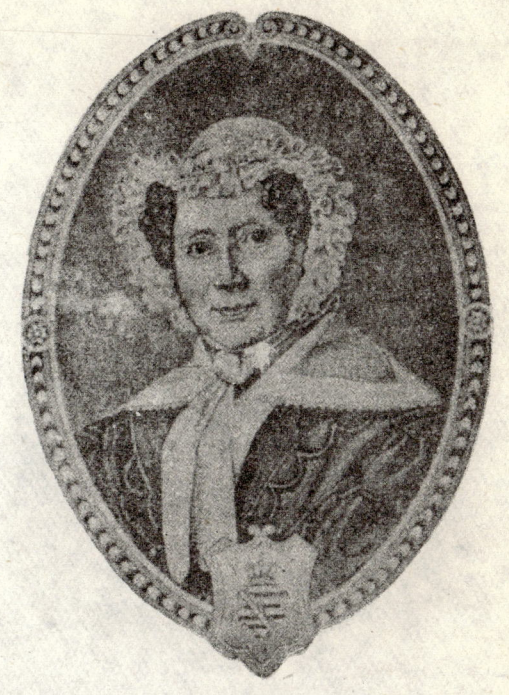

HAHNEMANN'S WIFE, HENRIETTE

See page 235 *Faces page 160*

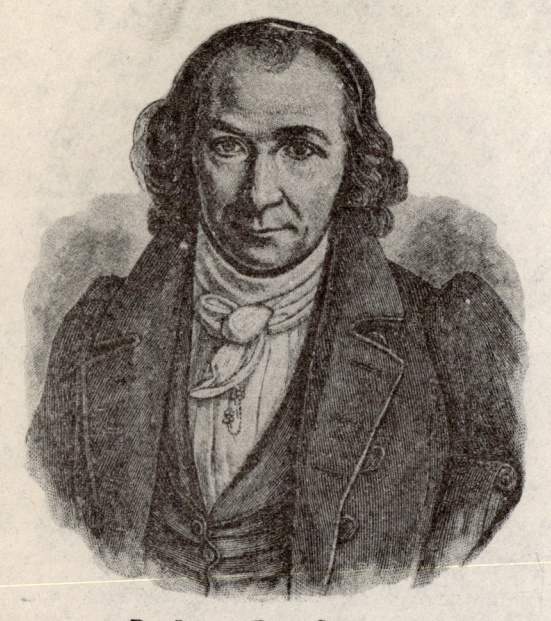

Dr. Johann Ernst Stapf

See page 183 *Faces page 161*

of the leading scientific journals, in the *Intelligenzblatt der Allgem. Literatur-Zeitung*, in Crell's *Chemical Annals*, and Scherer's *Journal of Chemistry*. It surely should have been evident that, just as thieves do not call in the civil authorities to inspect their robberies, neither do men of science invite inspection from scientific experts, if their wish is to palm off a common commodity for a rare one!

The first letter exposing his mistake simply demanded an explanation from Hahnemann as to how he was misled into offering at so high a price a substance which could be obtained for a few pennies. But from Professor Trommsdorff, an Erfurt apothecary, who had been one of the most appreciative among the reviewers of the *Apothecaries' Lexicon*, a direct attack on Dr. Hahnemann's integrity was forthcoming. It ended thus: "A great deal of impudence is required to pull the leg of the worthy German chemical fraternity and to defraud them of their money. . . . What will foreigners say to this story and what are the prospects of the past and future trustworthiness of Dr. Hahnemann?" In his eagerness to mingle scorn with a justifiable criticism, it is not hard to trace an antagonism to Hahnemann's new philosophy of medicine.

Professor Scherer, the editor of one of the three above-mentioned journals in which the announcement had appeared, staunchly defended Hahnemann, asking through the columns of his paper why Professor Trommsdorff had not awaited Hahnemann's defence before attacking him publicly in such a manner.

In Scherer's *Journal*, as well as in other papers, Hahnemann's answer appeared. In this reply he unreservedly admitted his error as regards the substance in question, adding: "I am incapable of wilfully deceiving; I may, however, like other men, be unintentionally mistaken. I am in the same boat with Klaproth and his 'diamond spar,' and with Proust and his 'pearl salt.'" He further exactly described the experiment which had led to his mistaken supposition.

At the end of 1804 Hahnemann found himself in Torgau, where he enjoyed a respite from his travels, remaining there for four years. Here the testing out of his method in practice only reassured him of the validity of his previous conclusions. His work as a translator also continued. To Steinacker, the publisher in Leipzig, he wrote in 1805 accepting his offer to bring out a translation of Albrecht von Haller's *Materia Medica of German Plants, together with their Economic and Technical Use*. In this work we find a translator's Introduction, in which Hahnemann writes: "I, the German translator, have no other merit on this occasion than that of handing over faithfully to my fellow-citizens this effort of incredible scholarship, this treasure of knowledge, exactly as it stands."

Just before this, Steinacker had published a small but significant work of Hahnemann's entitled *Æsculapius in the Balance*. Regarding this volume, we find the following in a postscript to the publisher: "Bring it especially before the notice of those who are not doctors. By so doing you will achieve a great purpose and prepare the way for a reform of the whole medical science—an event which must and will happen."

This essay touches upon many aspects of the subject which it sets out to discuss. The most important for us is its appeal against the laws whereby the Apothecaries' Guilds had been endowed with immense powers, through their monopoly of the right both to prepare and to dispense medicines.

Needless to say, the small amounts of the drug prescribed under homœopathy filled these people with apprehension, as this practice threatened the good fortune enjoyed under a regime which prescribed extravagantly. Hahnemann's use of simples instead of mixtures was again calculated inevitably to reduce their sales. Whilst one can sympathise with any trade or profession that sees its golden age waning before some advancement in science, Hahnemann's position, inspired as it was by the desire to render the greatest service to sick persons, was clearly essential. The situation which arose in this connection called forth in him such strong emotions and such disdainful glances at the developments in the history of prescribing that it seems best to let him speak for himself:

> "To fill to the brim the measure of deception and misapprehension attending the administration of medicine to the sick, the order of apothecaries was instituted—a guild which depends for existence on the complicated mixture of drugs. Never will the complicated formulæ cease to prevail as long as the powerful

order of apothecaries maintains its great influence. . . .

"Before these unhappy events the apothecaries were merely vendors of crude drugs, dealers in simples, druggists. . . . The physician bought only from those who had genuine and fresh materials, and mixed these for himself, according to his own fancy, but nobody prevented him from giving them to his patients in their simple and uncombined form. . . .

"The spirit of the advancing age had at length expunged from the list of drugs the pearls and jewels, the costly bezoar, the unicorn, and other things which were formerly so profitable to the apothecaries; simple processes for preparing the medicines were laid down; and the establishment of more stringent price regulations for the chemists threatened to convert their hitherto golden shops into silver ones, when things unobservedly took a turn more favourable to the apothecary and more disastrous to the art of medicine.

"The former medicinal laws, for example the *Constitutiones Frederici II Imperatoris*, had already begun to restrict the compounding of mixtures to the apothecaries, and thus in some measure to impose restrictions on the physicians. The more recent statutes completed the work by preventing physicians from converting the simple drugs into compound mixtures for themselves as well as forbidding them to give any medicine directly to the patients, and, as the expression was, 'to dispense.' Nothing could have been done better adapted to ruin the true art of medicine."

Hahnemann then refers to a book by Galen which treats of the adulteration of drugs and to deceptions practised by the apothecaries. This and other similar works, he tells us, constitute no small library.

We know that Hahnemann had no personal grounds for attacking the reputation of the apothecaries. His wife was the daughter of one, whilst her step-father, Häseler, had been the doctor's early associate in experimental chemistry. And had Hahnemann not given them the invaluable *Apothecaries' Lexicon*? It was rather the power accruing to their privileged position which he was assailing and their willingness to put this privilege before considerations relating to the cure of the sick. He drew attention to the dishonesty of some in the profession, only to shake the unqualified confidence reposed in them by law.

In England in the fourteenth century, many of them were foreigners, notably Italians and Germans. These various traders quarrelled much among themselves. They often charged each other with adulterating their wares. In the fifteenth century Letters Patents were granted to the Wardens of the Grocers' Company giving them the right of "garbling"—that is, separating and examining spices and drugs to prevent adulteration. Certain drugs had to be "officially garbled" before exposure for sale. The history of the word "garble" is interesting as illustrating that unreliability which Hahnemann was attacking. Derived from a late Latin word meaning "to sift," it passed very early into Arabic and also into Italian and Spanish. It means in effect to sort out. But men perceived that there was more than one kind of "sorting out" in practice, and hence we have our modern sense of "garbled" or "badly sorted."

Again protesting against the physicians being forbidden to prepare their own "instruments for the saving of life," Hahnemann continues:

"No human being could have fallen on such an idea a priori. It would have been much more sensible to prohibit authoritatively Titian, Guido Reni, Michael Angelo, Raphael, Correggio, or Mengs from preparing their own instruments (their expressive, beautiful, and durable colours) and to have ordered them to purchase them in some shop indicated. . . . And even had all their paintings become mere common market goods, the damage would not have been so great as if the life of even the meanest slave (for he too is a man) should be endangered by untrustworthy health instruments (medicines). . . . .

"Under these regulations, should there happen to be one single physician who should wisely wish to avoid that injudicious mode of prescribing multifarious mixtures of medicines and, for the weal of his patients and the furtherance of his art, should wish to prescribe simple medicines in their genuineness, he would be abused in every apothecary's shop until he abandoned a method that was so little profitable to the apothecaries, or else he must take his choice of either being harassed to death or of abandoning it and again writing compound prescriptions. In this case, what course would ninety-nine doctors out of a hundred choose? Do you know? I do! Therefore adieu to all progress in our art! Adieu to the successful treatment of the sick!"

These lines were written before or during Hähnemann's sojourn in Torgau, but they read like a record of an experience which awaited him even more acutely in the future. He was not only to become the physician who wished to dispense his own medicines, but the one historic figure in medicine at that time who insisted at all costs on doing so.

In the last passages, which form the concluding paragraphs of *Æsculapius in the Balance*, it will have been observed how the artist sympathies of the physician flash out again. A footnote reads: "I never heard of any great enamel painter who did not require to prepare his own colours, if he wished to have permanent brilliant colours and to produce masterpieces. . . ." Is he not here back again in memory in the workshops in Meissen? He may even have recollected that the "arcanists" or chemists had been the chief hindrance to his father's endeavours to advance the science and art of pottery.

The next work from the same pen was *The Organon of the Rational Art of Healing*, in which the subject matter is set out in short numbered sections. It is of the greatest importance as a concise survey of the whole field of homœopathic practice. Yet not only is it less readable than Hahnemann's Essays included in *Lesser Writings*, owing to its form, but, taken as a whole, it is also more definitely dependent upon insight derived from clinical experience.

Dr. August Bier, of Berlin University (whose tribute to homœopathy is summarised in the generous admission that, had he started his studies of its principles thirty years earlier, he would have been spared "a great many errors and détours") advises as follows:

> "Above all, I am of the opinion that no one should judge homœopathy, who has not tried homœopathic remedies or who has failed by reading to familiarise himself with the theory of homœopathy. I advise my colleagues who want to do the latter not to start with Hahnemann's writings but first to study the excellent work in two volumes by Haehl, *Samuel Hahnemann, his Life and Work*, and at least a few works by Hugo Schulz, and primarily the résumé of his teaching in his essays *Pharmaco-therapy* and *Similia Similibus curantur*."

He then names as the most practical German text-books two works by Stauffer: *Synopsis of Homœopathic Materia Medica* and *Homœotherapy*. For English-speaking readers may be added *Homœopathy Explained* by J. H. Clarke, M.D.; *The Case for Homœopathy* by C. E. Wheeler, M.D., B.S., B.Sc., and the *Materia Medica* by Dr. Neatby and Dr. Stonham. In recent years Dr. Bier has been instrumental in founding a Chair of Homœopathy in the Berlin University, the first to hold it being Dr. med. Ernst Bastanier.

The *Organon* went into several German editions. To the later editions Hahnemann prefixed the motto *Sapere Aude*, "Dare to be wise." These words from Horace we know had remained in his memory from boyhood, being inscribed to this day in three places in the Prince's School at Meissen.

On the title page of the first edition of the *Organon* Hahnemann also inscribed the following lines:

"Truth, for which all the eager world is fain,
Which makes us happy, lies for ever more
Not buried deep but lightly covered o'er
By the wise Hand that destined it for men."

These were taken from the writings of Gellert, who had preceded him at the Prince's School.

On the whole this much attacked physician, whose pen was indeed "the tongue of a ready speaker," if we may reverse the metaphor, was fortunate in obtaining the publication of his numerous works. But there were times when Hahnemann was uncertain of the co-operation of the publishers. On one occasion he wrote forcefully to his Dresden publisher Arnold:

"Freedom of action and liberty of the press must prevail, if great new truths are to be given to the world. What could Luther have done with his splendid ideas, if he had not been able to get them printed? if he could not have sent his out-spoken, plain truths hot from his heart to the press of his dear courageous friend, the bookseller and publisher Hans Luft, with all the hard words and abusive expressions he found useful for his object? Then everything was printed that was necessary, and it was only so, and in no other way, that the beneficial Reformation could be effected.... Hans Luft was almost as indispensable an instrument of the Reformation as Luther himself. I, too, require for the good cause (the much-needed reform of medicine) as warm and hearty a friend of truth for my publisher as Luft was for Luther."

Searching indeed were the thoughts concerning medical reform in Hahnemann's heart and mind, and not without good reason did he vex himself and his fellow-men with the question: "How does it happen that in thirty-five centuries since Æsculapius lived this so indispensable art of medicine has made so little progress?"

Increasingly at this time Torgau was being made the scene of military activities. At the command of Napoleon a large and formidable fortress was being built as a stronghold to defend the Elbe, and to keep the way open from Leipzig to Berlin and the East. Consequently, we find Hahnemann writing in January, 1811, to a friend, von Villers, a resident in the town of Göttingen:

"I am living, now nearly fifty-six years old, surrounded by my family, which is very dear to me—a wife of exceptional kindness and seven happy almost grown-up daughters...."

I am nearly always able to heal quickly and permanently any patients entrusted to my care, and in that way make many people happy, through the grace of Him Who made the remedies and put them into my hands. Am I not to be envied? But see, they are making all preparations to transmute Torgau into a big and terrible fortress in which my family is not likely to live in peace. I have to sell my dear and comfortable freehold house and move hence—undecided where."

At first it seems that thoughts of going to Göttingen were entertained, as Hahnemann felt a preference for a University town, but such were the restrictions laid upon the Senate and Professors there by the French Government that the idea was abandoned, in all probability for that reason. On September 28th in the same year von Villers received another letter: "Your letter gave a real day of festival to us—to me, who have now been living in Leipzig for four weeks, and to the whole of my family gathered round me." Again on December 3rd he wrote to Councillor Becker, who was still living in Gotha, revealing this migration of his from Torgau to Leipzig:

"I believe you do not know that I am six miles nearer to you. The *Mars constructor* was threatening to swallow me up amidst the gigantic ramparts of Torgau, and I escaped hitherwards. Nothing without God's dispensation! But I do regret the pretty house and the garden round it, where I think I have puzzled out many things for the good of man."

CHAPTER X

HAHNEMANN AND HIS CIRCLE

Leipzig, 1811-1820

In Leipzig Hahnemann now found himself for the third time. At the age of twenty as a student he had been there, and again at thirty-four, as a physician struggling with poverty and endeavouring to do as little positive injury as was possible under the existing methods of treatment. And now once more Hahnemann was there, seeking facilities as a teacher of the new method of treating the sick—similia similibus curantur—new, yet recognised here and there from the time of Hippocrates and not without its occasional demonstration in some historic cure, when used unwittingly by others. If we recall that it was to Leipzig that the youthful Christian Samuel Hahnemann was sent as a boy with a view to making a merchant of him, we must call this sojourn in Leipzig his fourth. But that was but a brief episode, indeed its significance lay in its brevity.

"The old world Leipzig of Samuel Hahnemann's day," writes Stephen Hobhouse, "has become a world city of busy and spacious thoroughfares. It is one of the greatest trading and manufacturing centres of Germany, and the whole German book-selling trade in particular is localised there in an extraordinarily well-organised way. The houses in which Hahnemann lived in Leipzig have either disappeared or been lost sight of. The University has been almost completely rebuilt and modernised, except for the Church, which is crowded against other buildings. It was interesting to read here of lectures, etc., still classified under the four mediæval 'Faculties': (1) Philosophy, including History, Languages and much else; (2) Medicine, including Veterinary degrees; (3) Jura, or Law; and (4) Theology.

"The statue of Hahnemann, not far off, appeared to me dignified and impressive; on a lofty pedestal in one of the busiest centres of city traffic, flanked by a grove of trees, surrounded by flower beds. It is very conspicuous and the seats round it were crowded. Its German inscription reads: '*To the Founder of Homœopathy, Samuel Hahnemann, born 1755, died 1843, from his grateful pupils and admirers.*'"

On settling down once more in this city the Saxon physician seems to have hoped that his house in the Burgstrasse, which bore the name of *Die Goldene Fahne*, or "The Golden Flag," might become a medical institute. This project did not mature. Hahnemann therefore applied for permission to lecture at the University. To this Rosenmüller, the Dean of the Medical Faculty, replied in February, 1812, that an external doctor could not obtain the right to deliver lectures until he had "defended his dissertation from the Upper Chair with a respondent" and had further deposited 50 thalers with the Faculty. If, on the other hand, these conditions were fulfilled the doctor could then advertise his lectures in the syllabus and announce them publicly.

Accordingly on June 26th in that summer Hahnemann delivered the oration required, and received the freedom to lecture at the University. This work is now included in his *Lesser Writings* under the title of *The Helleborism of the Ancients*. The subject of large and dangerous dosage had long held Hahnemann's imagination. Nor was their administration a matter of past history only. Hahnemann describes one treatment used in his day as "by no means inferior in severity to the helleborism of the ancient Greek and Roman physicians," adding: "such modes of treatment are not very unlike murders; the result alone (Nature having given the fortunate turn to the case) renders them uncriminal, and almost imparts to them the lustre of a good action, the saving of life." Then follows the eminently characteristic reflection: "This cannot be the divine art, which like the mighty workings of Nature should effect the greatest deeds simply, mildly, and unobservedly by means of the smallest agencies."

As far back as 1796 Hahnemann wrote: "White Hellebore, an incomparable drug, produces the most poisonous effects, which can inspire the doctor striving for perfection with caution, and with the hope that he may overcome some of the severest cases of disease which have hitherto remained without help." He was able to write thus only because he had even then sensed the need of reducing the power for harm (and correspondingly increasing the power for cure) by diminishing his doses to a degree unheard of in his time. The doctrine that the greater the poison the severer the malady that it could eradicate, if rightly potentised, was also with Hahnemann a fully accepted axiom. In the remarks which he prefixed to his later proving of Helleborus Niger, he states: "I myself gathered the root which I used for my trials, and hence am convinced of its genuineness."

A letter from Dr. Huck, a physician who was present at the delivery of Hahnemann's paper, expressed unqualified praise.

"To hear Hahnemann, the keenest and boldest investigator of Nature, deliver a masterpiece of his intellect and industry, was to me a truly beatific enjoyment. . . . He will deliver his private lectures at Michaelmas. I shall be a student next year again and, if exceptional circumstances do not prevent it, I will see what I can derive from this wonderful source. The strongest of his opponents were so courteous as to acknowledge that they were wholly of his opinion, medically speaking, and they thought that if anyone wished to say anything he would be obliged to discuss the matter philologically. He covered himself with renown."

A sense of rest is produced upon the mind by the fact that even "opponents" on this occasion showed courtesy.

As regards philological enquiry, we know that Hahnemann welcomed this. With Professor Adam Beyer, who was then a research worker in languages at Leipzig, Hahnemann met at times for the discussion of syntactical and advanced subjects of criticism in Latin and Greek philology. Professor Franz Albrecht, Seminary Director in Köthen, a personal friend of Hahnemann's for many years, to whom we owe this information, adds that "the Leipzig Professor paid great attention to his medical friend's opinion in any philological controversy." Principal Albrecht remarks with some surprise that this love of ancient philology had not suffered, as it might well have done, from Hahnemann's wide knowledge of modern languages and the continuous work of translations from them upon which he had been engaged.

A circle of medical students now gathered round the new lecturer. That it was small, no doubt was a disappointment to Hahnemann, though judging by the evidence of one of his most devoted disciples he went out of his way to decry current methods when he might well have limited himself to the advocacy of his own. This naturally antagonised Dr. Rosenmüller and Dr. Clarus, the clinical Professor, who became not only an enemy to all that Hahnemann taught, but also in some measure a persecutor of any who chose to become his followers. As the latter could by virtue of the office he held as the highest medical authority in Saxony appear as Prosecutor and Judge, Hahnemann's attitude promised no good to himself, especially as it was his desire and need to dispense his own medicines—a practice against the existing law, as narrowly interpreted.

Whether in his lectures Hahnemann was carried away as he had so often been before by a picture of the needless additional sufferings of those who were put through the round of venesection, drastic purgings and emetics, not to mention the over-drugging, or whether new occasions for a more personal irritation arose to account at least partly for this seeming invitation to self-defeat, it is hard to surmise.

Yet however much even his followers may have been justified in regretting the torrents of condemnation which Hahnemann heaped upon orthodox medicine, it is conceivable that, had he gone to the other extreme and adopted a purely conciliatory tone, his following would have included men of a very different stamp. Consequently, his group, though larger in his day, would probably have dwindled after he was gone by virtue of its own indecision. As it was, the few who rallied round this teacher were students and doctors with sufficient penetration to see below the turbulent outpourings of indignation to the permanent nature of Hahnemann's contribution to medicine. They became keen fellow-workers and remained faithful over long years, and after his death carried forward his work.

Of Hahnemann's personal relations with his followers, Dr. Franz Hartmann (his critic as well as disciple) gives us a pleasing insight:

"We often had an opportunity of admiring the amiability with which he charmed us all when we made part of his family. There sat the silver-haired old man, with his high arched brow, his bright piercing eyes and calm searching countenance, in the midst of us and of his own children, who likewise participated in those evening entertainments. Here he showed plainly that the serious exterior which he exhibited in every-day life belonged only to his deep and constant search after the goal which he had set himself, but was in no respect the mirror of his interior, the bright side of which so readily unfolded itself on suitable occasions in its fairest light. The mirthful humour, the familiarity and openness, the wit that he displayed were alike engaging.

"How comfortable the Master felt in the circle of his beloved and his friends, among whom he numbered not only his pupils, but also the learned of other faculties, who did homage to his learning; how beneficial was the recreation which he then allowed himself after eight o'clock in the evening, seated in his armchair wearing his velvet cap and dressing gown, with a glass of Leipzig white beer and his pipe. . . . He liked to converse specially on objects of the natural sciences or on conditions of foreign countries and their inhabitants, and he appeared displeased when in these hours his advice was sought with regard to cases of disease. He was then either laconic, or called out to the enquirer in a friendly way, 'to-morrow on this subject.' He would often during his consulting hours on the following day refer to the question raised, and stood by with his kind advice. He liked to see people express their opinion openly, even if they contradicted him, and occasionally he would surrender his opinion to that of his opponent."

To his impressions Hartmann adds a description of the "suppers" which once or twice a year were given at the doctor's house in Burgstrasse. To these none were invited but those who had

"distinguished themselves through diligence, intelligence and strict morality. . . . During these supper parties things were not altogether homœopathic, for although I can vouch for a perfect simplicity of the food served, yet instead of white beer a good wine was provided, of which, however, out of deference to the Master, only a moderate amount was consumed. . . . Joyous humour and wit dominated these gatherings, and the desire to laugh was unending, for as a rule other talented men were invited. Here Hahnemann was the most cheerful man. . . . When the meal was ended, a pipe was smoked and about 11 o'clock the gathering dispersed."

Whether Hahnemann was still smoking the pipe preserved in the dining room of the picturesque old tavern in Meissen, kept now by Herr Vincent Richter, cannot be known, but there an old well-worn pipe lies with a small imprint of Hahnemann on it and a presentation inscription with the date 1790, alongside the coloured "rebus" which we have described in an earlier chapter. The room is fitted up as a sort of local museum, and its treasures were collected by the present host's father, though nothing is recorded of how either the pipe or rebus came to be in it.

"The inn," wrote the same recent English visitor to Meissen whom we have quoted already, "stands close under the old Frauenkirche. I went in and drank a glass of unfermented grape juice—*frische Most*. As I left—a charming scene—a large cart was before the door with casks full of dark blue grapes, which men were carrying in to press for 'Most.' The cart and casks were decorated with vine leaves." "The pipe," the letter continues, "shows evidence of much use, presumably it was enjoyed by Hahnemann. As Dr. Preuss says, one would not give such a present to a *Griesgram*—a morose old chap!"

Preuss uses this and still more the picture rhyme with its childlike happiness, its spice of golden humour and playfulness, to stress the error of the popular over-emphasis put by some on the atmosphere of suspicion, unsociability and gloom engendered in Hahnemann by his fight against persecution. He thinks the memory of Hahnemann suffers unjustly from his reputation in this respect.

This glimpse of the grape traders reminds us that in the year of the presentation of the pipe, 1790 (also the year of the cinchona experiment), Hahnemann had translated Fabbroni's *Art of making Wine in accordance with sensible Principles* from the Italian, with annotations. Hartmann has commented on the moderation enjoined by the hospitable doctor at his supper parties, and we find Hahnemann writing in the year with which our present chapter opens to his friend von Villers, "I cannot recommend the frequent use of wine unless it be mixed with water, as was the custom of the Romans and the Greeks." In a conversation with a friend of his, the Rev. T. Everest, who questioned him on the subject, Hahnemann referred to his smoking as a "useless habit acquired in earlier days when I had to sit up every other night to earn bread for my children whilst I pursued my own researches during the day." This was especially in the Stötteritz days. Mr. Everest, the Rector of a Gloucestershire parish, was a convinced homœopath and later both preached and published a sermon on behalf of the Hahnemann Hospital in London.

His consultations were from nine to twelve in the morning and from two to four in the afternoon. "No person was permitted to enter the hall who had not first passed the review, which was performed every week alternately by one of his daughters, and for which she placed herself like a warder at a little window next the hall door."

His apartment was usually filled with patients. He examined accurately and wrote down in his journal himself all the symptoms of which the patient complained, even those apparently insignificant, and referred to them one after the other previous to furnishing the medicine required. This was obtained from another room. After the clock had struck twelve in the morning and four in the afternoon no visit from any quarter was received. At twelve to the minute he was called to dinner, after which his attention was not easily directed to anything else. At one time, in the warmth of conversation, having twice disregarded the call, at the third more earnest call from his wife, he smilingly observed, "This time I shall get a dark look." "This expression," Hartmann adds, "several times heard from him convinced me that this great man, who had so much influence over others, had to be placed under a guardian in his own house, which, however, he willingly endured. . ."

Karl Hornburg, a friend of his childhood, had first introduced Franz Hartmann to the Doctor. They shared rooms and Hartmann soon followed the example of his friend, who six months after his entrance to the University changed theology for medicine. Of the two Hartmann proved himself the most assiduous in his studies, and his help was sought for later in connection with the *Archiv*, of which Dr. Stapf was the editor. He is known also as a disciple of Jacob Boehme, the Silesian mystic of the seventeenth century.

At Leipzig, from the year 1806, Stapf himself had been chiefly under the tuition of Drs. Clarus and Rosenmuller at the University, so that it is certain that nothing in the teaching he had received there had predisposed him to a study of homœopathy. The history of medicine claimed his interest keenly, and before taking his degree he had withdrawn to practice. In after years, writing of himself as if about another, under the name of *Philalethes*, he reveals something of the same dissatisfaction that had oppressed Hahnemann.

"Philalethes pursuing the paths of others faithfully as he did his own, he still nowhere found what he desired and what would satisfy. Everywhere he encountered that unmistakable lack of a more sublime, a more natural unity, of that harmony between theory and practice which I should like to call natural balance.... It was painful and disturbing to him to meet so much that sounded learned and yet was ridiculous and unnatural and in spite of all his strivings he found himself more and more hopelessly distant from the desired goal.... He was almost abandoning so strangely cultivated a field and devoting himself exclusively to the study of other natural sciences (particularly to chemistry, which he always preferred) as these were evidently far in advance of medicine in their development. Then, in 1812, a propitious fate brought *The Organon of the Rational Art of Healing*, by Samuel Hahnemann, into his hands."

Curiously enough another work of Hahnemann's relating to his discovery, *Fragmenta de Viribus*, published in 1805, had been in Stapf's library almost unheeded for years. It contained the words "Nemo me melius novit, quam manca sint et tenuia"—"Nobody knows better than I how imperfect and insufficient it all is." Yet in Hufeland's *Bibliothek* the essay is described as "uncommonly interesting and creditable." The work contained the first collection of remedies which had been "proved" on a healthy subject. The value of its contribution to medical thought, Dr. Stapf acknowledges, had escaped him. Even the reading of the *Organon* was undertaken many times with "a lively scepticism." Not content to give only thought to the subject, where thought alone was inadequate, Stapf put the new propositions into practice, with the result that he was able to declare that the work withstood the most assiduous tests that he could devise. The following year Stapf got into touch with Hahnemann, from which time a long friendship and co-operation in the once almost abandoned medical field persisted. Stapf's description of his wanderings in the wilderness could indeed, as we have hinted, read as Hahnemann's own, with just this difference, that they covered a shorter period and were not attended with such difficulties in personal life as the years through which Hahnemann had to toil. There is therefore not the same anguish in them that we find in such a letter as that which Hahnemann wrote to Hufeland.

In June of this year 1813, Stapf passed his Bachelor's examination, and, early in the year following, his *rigorosum*. By April he gave his Doctor's "dissertation." The son of the first Rector of the Maria Magdalena Church in Naumburg, he made his native town the scene of his practice.

It was soon after that Doctor Stapf received

from Hahnemann what appears to be almost his only recorded pronouncement on the political situation of the time, yet the doctor, we know, especially missed the reading of the political papers, if pressure of work forbade their perusal. Moreover, a strong political sense was evidenced in his concern for bringing about happier conditions in the cities of Germany. This was contained in a letter to his new colleague and disciple and more than echoes a note of hope which had evidently been struck previously by Stapf himself.

"I am entirely of your opinion that the times will soon be better. In our previous state of subjugation, everybody was silent, especially the good people. The better minds had been so intimidated and disheartened that they did not dare to express their feelings. Only the voice of the common mob was heard, glad in the general depravity to be able to give its evil tendencies full play, and to be able to suppress the best in speech and writing, as exemplified by the suppressor of all [Napoleon]. The literary rabble alone raised its head in the last decade and tried to overthrow and annihilate everything that had a nobler and more broadminded tendency. But now, as the spirit of our venerable ancestors—heroic courage, resolution, faithfulness, friendship, honesty of purpose, humanity and love of truth and of man's happiness—seems to be reawakening among the guardians of the peoples, . . . Truth will once more ascend the throne and that which is good will no longer be derisively misunderstood."

These penetrating observations were followed a few months after by a letter to the same friend containing the ejaculation: "If this wicked war would only leave us in peace, so that we might again be able to print something! Then we might take a new lease of life."

As the proving of drugs on the healthy in order to elucidate symptoms they could call forth was an essential factor in Hahnemann's method, a band of "provers" was formed—that is, of persons willing to test drugs on themselves. The "Provers' Union" engaged in this difficult and important work formed the nucleus of Hahnemann's later corporate experiments in proving. It included the names of Stapf, Gross, Hornburg, Franz, Wislicensus, Teuthorn, Herrmann, Rückert, Langhammer, Hartmann, and Hahnemann himself.

"These, the first pupils and adherents of Hahnemann," writes Hartmann, "were bound very closely to the master. . . . Franz, who had been cured by Hahnemann of a very serious disease, was older than the others, and was his assistant. He was a good botanist and collected plants. When they were in Hahnemann's collection, then no time was lost in preparing them as fast as possible for medicinal use. Both then laboured with diligence, and Franz also arranged the symptoms of the provings, according to the scheme of Hahnemann, copying them many times."

We are told further by this disciple that "no one was ashamed to perform the humblest labour; the chemical laboratory was a sanctum from which we were as difficult to drive as a fox from his burrow."

Of the first provers, Dr. Rückert in after years assisted Hahnemann in preparing a repertory to his last important work. Dr. Gross, who was a pastor's son, was of very especial assistance to Hahnemann in the proving of drugs because of his extraordinarily developed faculty for fine observation. He was also later the writer of a *Dietetic Handbook for the Healthy and the Sick*, and another essay entitled *Directions for the Mother and Child*. That he contributed a work on the second subject is not surprising, since, as a member of the group of "provers," Gross first made experiments with chamomilla, which all who practice homœopathy have found invaluable in many of the difficulties of early life.

A trained doctor himself, there are no indications that Hahnemann undervalued the co-operation of trained minds. As we shall see later, his small but enthusiastic circle of adherents were drawn almost entirely from his professional colleagues or medical students. There were, it is true, exceptions, amongst whom his friend Carl von Bönninghausen was one, a man of varied and wide attainments, who became a celebrated practitioner. It is clear that he regarded a laity, enlightened on the broad principles of medical work and its history, as a likely incentive to the profession to which he belonged to improve its art.

As illustrating the type of man whom the new system of medicine and its founder could attract, and with whom Hahnemann enjoyed a long and deep friendship, a sketch of Bönninghausen may be given. Born of an old but none too prosperous family of the Prussian nobility, at the age of eighteen he went to the University of Groningen for three years, taking the doctorate in law in 1806, after which he went almost immediately to the Bar. As a student he had attended lectures on medicine and the natural sciences. Bönninghausen in 1807 accompanied his father to the court of Louis Bonaparte, then King of Holland, and obtained a position at the Court. When after three years Louis Bonaparte abdicated he devoted himself to agriculture and its subsidiary sciences, having, like Hahnemann, a special interest in botany. Two years later he became Landrat (Sheriff) for the district of Coesfeld, and remained in that office until he was appointed General Commissioner of the land register of the Rhineland and Westphalia, which had only recently been drawn up. He published a work on the similarity between the flora of the Rhine and Westphalia and that of England, drawing attention to their resemblance in 1824. Following this he was made Director of the Botanical Gardens in Münster.

In 1827 Bönninghausen was overtaken with a serious illness, and when, early in the year following, he wrote to a physician who was also one of his botanical friends, Dr. Werke of Herford, it was to say farewell to him, all hope of recovery being abandoned. Werke, unbeknown to his friend, had now become a convinced homœopath and immediately prescribed for Bönninghausen. A marked improvement occurred, and by the end of the summer Bönninghausen was himself again. It was later, when he had himself acquired fame in the effecting of cures, that doctors from France, Holland and America came to Münster to see him, and to learn from him the secret of his efficiency in the healing art. Bönninghausen now sought official permission to practise, and in July, 1843, he was granted authority to do so by order of the Cabinet of King Friedrich Wilhelm IV without undergoing medical examination.

Bönninghausen's practical answer to the charge made that homœopathy was a mere covering for faith-cure was a very considerable practice amongst animals. In this sphere of veterinary medicine, in which "faith" could not be accredited to the patients, he met with equal success. Some years later it was Bönninghausen who arranged for an annual meeting of homœopathic physicians in Westphalia and the Rhineland, and he lived to receive the title of "Doctor of Medicine" from the Cleveland Homœopathic Medical College in the United States. He was further appointed Knight of the Legion of Honour on April 20th, 1861, by the Emperor Napoleon III. That this was in association with his widely spread distinction as a healer of the sick we need not doubt, as there is evidence that he was some years earlier in medical attendance on the Empress Eugénie. A Prussian newspaper at the time observed: "This physician, equally distinguished as a practitioner and as a writer, was originally a layman and as such was early declared by Hahnemann to be his most excellent student." Carl von Bönninghausen's *Lesser Writings* are of peculiar value as being the outcome of this intimate tuition at the fountain-head of research and discovery. "Surely," he writes with regard to the infinitesimal in this collection of his works, "Aristotle is right when he says: 'Ignorance can only attain to science through the knowledge of what is wonderful and incredible in nature.'"

In citing Bönninghausen as a "lay physician" we must note that he had attended medical lectures and had made an intensive study of plants, and also remind ourselves of the differences between those days and our own. At that time, it will be remembered, it was possible for an undergraduate like Hahnemann, after leaving Vienna, to be recommended as physician to the household of the Governor of Transylvania with freedom to practise in the district by no less an authority than the Rector of the Vienna University.

Of the method of "proving" adopted, Hahnemann himself tells us:

"I gave the medicines prepared by myself for this purpose in higher or lower dynamizations, in larger or smaller doses, as everyone could take them without being too exhausted... The chief thing was, always to see that the provers should be free from erroneous diet and mode of living, as healthy as possible, and keen to explore the high truths which we are expecting to find, with a strong sense of conscientious honesty, without expecting the slightest worldly advantage, not even to hope for the honour of being publicly mentioned as a 'prover.'"

Severe criticisms met the work, which was condemned on the ground of its danger to those who subjected themselves to experiment. The year before Hahnemann left Torgau a review in a medical paper of the *Organon* (which gives in some of its sections directions for provers) strongly denounced the proceeding as unpermissible. Even if it must be conceded that some danger still remained after the most careful precautions were taken, it is surely true that those who are in health should at least be the best able to bear the risk. Thomas Fuller, the seventeenth century divine, wrote of "The Good Physician":

"He hansels not his new experiments on the bodies of his patients; letting loose mad receipts into the sick man's body to try how well Nature in him will fight against them, while he himself stands by and sees the battle; except it be in desperate cases when death must be expelled by death."

It is from the recollections of the Baron Ernst von Brunnow, whom Hahnemann had the happiness of setting free from an ailing condition which had beset him from childhood, that we have a closer opportunity of judging of the extent to which Hahnemann was able to eliminate the harmful factors in his practical demonstration of drug-action. He tells us that "a very peculiar mode of life prevailed in Hahnemann's household at Leipzig. The members of the family, the University students and the patients all lived for one idea, the promotion of homœopathy. The four grown-up daughters assisted their father in the preparation of medicines and with the students eagerly took part in the provings." To these remarks he adds: "That these carefully instituted provings were not at all injurious to any of them, I can personally testify from my own experience when I lived amongst them." We know also that one of Hahnemann's sons was a keen "prover." The precautionary measures which Hahnemann took as prover included a careful study of "antidotes" to all the drugs used, and the keeping of these to hand.

It is of interest that Dr. Stapf tested upon himself thirty-two medical substances, whilst Hahnemann in the course of years proved in his own person no fewer than a hundred.

"For years, for half a lifetime," writes Dr. Tyler of this heroic band of investigators, "they had been 'proving' drug after drug, and suffering its effects in their own minds and bodies. Naturally they had less difficulty in recognising a personally experienced drug-picture in a patient. It had been branded on their memories by suffering. The greatest ability to help is achieved ever at the greatest cost."

CHAPTER XI

THE LEIPZIG APOTHECARIES

Leipzig and Köthen, 1820-1821

THE daily walks of the Hahnemann family at this time, which were sometimes extended to Schleuzig or Gohlis, are sketched by von Brunnow's pen:

"It was on a clear spring day . . . that I, a young, newly-enrolled student of law, sauntered with some of my companions along the cheerful promenade of Leipzig. Among the teachers of the University were to be found many notables and not a few originals. Many a professor and master stalked gravely along in the old-fashioned dress of the former century, with peruque and bag, silk stockings, and buckles on his shoes, while the pampered sons of the landed gentry swaggered about in Hussar jackets and pantaloons ornamented with points, or in leather breeches, with high Dragoon boots and clinking spurs. . . . 'Tell me,' said I to an older student than myself, who was walking with me, 'who is that old gentleman with so extraordinarily intelligent a countenance, who walks respectfully arm-in-arm with his somewhat corpulent spouse, and is followed by two pairs of rosy girls?' 'That is the celebrated Dr. Hahnemann. He takes a walk regularly every afternoon with his wife and daughters,' was the reply. 'What,' rejoined I, 'is there about this Hahnemann that makes him celebrated?' 'Why, he is the discoverer of the homœopathic system of medicine, which is turning old medicine topsy-turvy,' replied my acquaintance, who, like myself, was from Dresden, and had also enlisted himself under the colours of Themis."

The pen of this law-student has described how, "after the day had been spent in labour, Hahnemann was in the habit of recruiting himself from eight to ten o'clock by conversation with his circle of trusty friends. All his friends and scholars then had access to him, and in the middle of the whispering circle the old Æsculapius reclined in a comfortable armchair."

"Although living in luxurious and elegant Leipzig, Dr. Hahnemann's daughters took no part in any public amusement, and were clad in the simplest fashion and undertook most cheerfully the humblest household services." "Hahnemann," he continues, "at that time was in his sixty-second year. Locks of silver-white clustered round his high and thoughtful brow, from under which his animated eyes shone with piercing brilliancy. His whole countenance had a quiet, searching, grand expression; only rarely did a gleam of fine humour play over the deep earnestness, which told of the many sorrows and conflicts endured. His carriage was upright, his step firm, his motions lively as those of a man of thirty. When he went out his dress was the simplest; a dark coat, with short small-clothes and stockings. But in his room at home he preferred the old household, gaily-figured, dressing gown, the yellow stockings and the black velvet cap. The long pipe was seldom out of his hand, and smoking was the only infraction he allowed himself to commit upon his severe rules of regimen. His drink was water, milk, or white beer; his food of the most frugal sort. The whole of his domestic economy was as simple as his dress. Instead of a writing desk he used nothing but a large plain deal table, upon which there constantly lay three or four enormous folios, in which he had written the history of the cases of his patients, and which he used diligently to turn up and write in while conversing with them."

As one of the most serious symptoms in von Brunnow's case had been the effect of his ill-health upon his eyes, it can be imagined with what gratitude he experienced his recovery during the days of his studentship when good sight for the purposes of studying was so essential. As an expression of his indebtedness to Hahnemann, the law student, having passed his examination and entered into the State service, began to read French medical writings in order to familiarise himself with the technical terms needed in order to translate the *Organon of the Rational Art of Healing* into that language. This project met with Hahnemann's approval, and when accomplished not only did von Brunnow's translation do a great deal to advance a knowledge of Hahnemann's method of treatment in France, but also led to its study in Italy, England, Hungary, Poland and Russia. Physicians in these countries corresponded with von Brunnow, a fact which stimulated his own enthusiasm even more.

Into Hahnemann's daily round there was now brought a patient of European importance, Prince Schwarzenberg, the Field Marshal who had commanded the allied armies against Napoleon. The advice given to Schwarzenberg to seek the help of the Saxon doctor came from one of his own two Court physicians in Austria. Accordingly, as Hahnemann would not leave his own practice, the General, ill as he was, travelled to Leipzig and made his home on an estate outside the city, to which Hahnemann was driven.

It was in May of 1820 that Goethe, observing events in the medical world, wrote from Karlsbad:

> "In this place a curious game is being played by refusing and damming up innovations of every kind, *e.g.* it is forbidden to cure by magnetism, and nobody is allowed to practise by Hahnemann's method. . . . But now Prince Schwarzenberg, very ill and probably incurable, has confidence in this new Theophrastus Paracelsus and begs for leave of absence from the Emperor to seek a cure across the border."

THE LEIPZIG APOTHECARIES

The fact that this permission was granted by the Emperor Francis I, who only the previous year had issued a decree against homœopathy under pressure from his medical adviser, von Stifft, had a touch of humour which could hardly have escaped the imagination of a poet and dramatist.

But even the continuance of General Schwarzenberg's important consultations was threatened by the fact that the apothecaries of Leipzig had determined to prevent Hahnemann from preparing and himself giving to his patients the remedies used. To support themselves in their desire to hinder and even make impossible his work, they brought forward the decrees against a physician so acting.

Fearing lest freedom to pursue the course of treatment which he was trying as a last resort should abruptly come to an end, Schwarzenberg on July 20th appealed to the King of Saxony through his government. He wrote:

"The rumour which is being circulated here, that Dr. Hahnemann will be forbidden the practice of his method of treatment by an act of the Government, forces upon me the necessity to beg His Majesty the King to graciously grant an audience to my Adjutant General, the Colonel Baron Wernhardt, so that he may put before him some information regarding this new method of treatment which I am undergoing at present. . . . Since I have been under Dr. Hahnemann's treatment some of my attacks have already been alleviated. . . ."

Schwartzenberg's intermediary, writing a few days later, explained that various applications had been made both for and against Hahnemann's position regarding self-dispensing, and stated that owing to General Schwarzenberg's letter the Government of the country had considered it necessary to bring the matter for final decision before the King himself, which was being done on the following day.

After this appeal had been lodged the King of Saxony, who was cousin to the General, wrote:

> "The Colonel Baron von Wernhardt has already delivered your message to me in connection with the matter of Dr. Hahnemann of Leipzig, and has received from me an answer to the effect that I shall make enquiries. I have ordered all that is necessary to be done, and arranged at the same time that no further steps shall be taken against Dr. Hahnemann..."

The above letter from Schwarzenberg to the King of Saxony shows that there was improvement at first.

> "The first consequence of this honourable tribute to Hahnemann," von Brunnow observes, "was the suspension of the process the apothecaries had commenced against him. Had Prince Schwarzenberg recovered, then would homœopathy have enjoyed an immediate triumph in Saxony, and even in all Germany; but every art has its limits. Hahnemann undertook the case as a desperate one on which he could try the effects of homœopathy.

To the astonishment of all, the patient felt himself better from day to day, and he was seen driving about after a little time; but the powers of life had been too much weakened to permit of his recovery. The former malady returned, and the Field Marshal died on October 15th, 1820, in the same town into which, in the same month of the year in 1813, he had entered as conqueror. Although the post-mortem proved that no medical skill could by any possibility have been successful in the case, yet the issue of it was very injurious to Hahnemann. The suspended process was immediately resumed, and it was decided that Hahnemann must give up dispensing his own medicines."

Brunnow here refers to a law-suit which had early that year been entered against Hahnemann by the apothecaries, the charge being that he and his pupils were "entrenching on their privileges." As a result, Hahnemann had been brought before the court. At the close of the hearing he stated his intention of handing in a "written deposition to precede the final judgment." This long and carefully-reasoned document appears in Haehl's biography under the title, *Remonstrance with the Apothecaries of Leipzig* (see Supplement 63).

It is enough to assure us of Hahnemann's sense of duty fulfilled, as far as opportunity had offered, that he attended the funeral of the Prince, walking on foot in the procession and taking calmly the jibes and occasional hissing which an ignorant crowd meted out to this butt of professional criticism. The document recording the cause of death as apoplexy was signed and sealed by four physicians, including the names of both Hahnemann and his most bitter opponent, Dr. Clarus.

It is not without interest that Goethe reveals in various places in his writings his awareness not only of the evils in the medical profession, but also of the reforms that were brooding, and of the light that was already spreading in the direction of treatment by "likes" and by small doses. Thus Faust, walking on the outskirts of a town, speaks with his assistant of the greater havoc wrought amongst the patients by the treatment than by the pestilence. Again, in a later passage:

"Whatever the disease, 'tis like to like
Forms the great secret of the healing art."

These utterances in themselves do not require us to assume that the poet was committed to Hahnemann's principle; but of the fact that he studied it and held its advocate in high regard there is evidence. In a letter dated 13th September, 1820, from Jena, Goethe wrote: "With many thanks I am returning the MS. [of Dr. Hahnemann] lent to me and I have given a copy to a reliable doctor. Next winter it will give us an opportunity . . . of thinking with pleasure of the wonder-physician."

Following the widely observed event of Schwarzenberg's death, an attack was made on Hahnemann by thirteen Leipzig physicians. The opposition of "the thirteen" did not, however, centre round this case, though no doubt they found in the feeling which the General's death produced a favourable atmosphere for its propagation. Over a number of years Hahnemann had, as we have seen, from time to time to appeal against the application of his prescription for scarlet fever, belladonna, to "purpura miliaris" (for this he had prescribed aconite). Recently, again, he had issued publicly, for the benefit of the inhabitants of Leipzig, an opposing diagnosis of an eruptive fever which had been prevailing. This had angered the professional pride of his colleagues, and their expression of annoyance had included even a denial that the use of belladonna as a preventive in scarlet fever could be claimed as a discovery by Hahnemann. We have already referred to Hufeland's work published in favour of its use as a prophylactic and remedy, and to the fact that he readily ascribed its discovery to none other but Hahnemann.

The statement of "the thirteen" appeared in a public journal, the *Leipziger Zeitung*, and a few days later Hahnemann replied. His "defence" revealed clearly that this incident in medical controversy represented a far wider line of attack than was apparent at a glance:

"There stand thirteen gentlemen," he wrote, "colleagues of mine in this town, who are struggling hard to show readers, here and elsewhere, how very vexed they are at my reputation (such as it is), at my discoveries, at my writings (which they will not take upon themselves to read), and at the cures which, by the grace of God, I have successfully effected on patients abandoned by the doctors, whereby I have gained the love and esteem of this community and others."

When we add to the medical ostracism the renewed opposition of the apothecaries on the question of self-dispensing, a privilege which Hahnemann esteemed as essential to his work, it will be appreciated that this seriously counterbalanced the joy of having an increasing number of patients loyal through cures experienced, besides a band of enthusiastic students, and the following of individual physicians of wide intellectual outlook who were not afraid to investigate the new method closely for themselves.

It was indeed obviously the intention of his opponents so to heighten his discomfort that Hahnemann would be compelled to bestir himself once more to seek another sphere for his work. The apothecaries had a stronger weapon than a psychological one. The law existing against self-dispensing, at least as they chose to interpret it, was on their side.

When it is remembered that Hahnemann only administered medicines as simples and in potency, all this talk of the "law" relating to his dispensing them becomes absurd, a mere battle over a legal fiction. To be on the losing side, nevertheless, meant to the doctor the whole difference between freedom to serve his fellows in the light that had broken in upon his mind, and absolute defeat.

Keen and prolonged over many years were the

conflicts in which the doctor was engaged. Nevertheless the larger sympathies of his life rang true to a surprising degree, and there are recurrent indications that Hahnemann recognised the weakness of a vindictive spirit. It was his pen that had written to an old friend:

> "He who, as regards vexations about injuries, does not remain master of himself, does not treat them with indifference, but allows his mind to be embittered, poisoned by them, will not live long; he will so soon have to leave this world. And what an odious thing it is to be overcome with anger! Try to keep from you all sensitiveness in regard to such things so that nothing can deprive you of your composure, of your God-given tranquillity. Take warning, learn this beautiful lesson! It will do you good."

No man who had not both failed and attained as regards this gift of self-mastery could have written such counsel to another.

In 1820 Professor Lindner, a friend of Hahnemann's at the Leipzig University, had published a "Defence of the Homœopathic Method of Healing . . . confirmed by attested and striking facts—by a layman for doctors and lay people." This was a reply to the criticism by Professor Puchelt, a strong opponent of Hahnemann's method, though an opponent who could also oppose those who attacked homœopathy in an unworthy manner. To Professor Lindner we owe also a sidelight on these difficult times, showing in what measure the townsfolk of Leipzig felt themselves involved in this feud in the medical world. "On the attempt being made by the apothecaries and several doctors to drive Dr. Hahnemann by force out of Leipzig," he tells us, "Dr. Volkmann, Town Clerk of Leipzig, determined to enter a protest against it at the Appeal Court of Dresden." This appeal was signed by Professor Lindner himself and forty other citizens and sent in to Dresden. . . . The result was that Hahnemann's position was reconsidered by the authorities and he was able to remain in Leipzig until the way for his departure opened.

As a Mason he had joined the Leipzig lodge "Minerva of the Three Palms," and to a fellow-mason, Dr. Billig of Altenburg, he had written:

> "I only wish to settle in some country or village where the post may facilitate my connection with distant parts, and where I may not be annoyed by the presumption of any apothecary; because, as you know, the pure practice of this art can only employ such minute weapons, such small doses of medicine, that no apothecary can supply them profitably. And owing to the mode in which he has learnt and has always carried on his business, an apothecary could not help finding the whole affair ridiculous, and would ridicule it to the public and to the patients. Therefore it would be impossible for this and for other reasons to find an assistant in the ordinary apothecary for the practice of homœopathy."

With his use of high potencies it would indeed have been impossible for Hahnemann to place their preparation in the hands of those who had not even the remotest respect for his method, and who might easily have been tempted to think that such inconceivably small quantities were altogether negligible. They might have even supplied nothing but the diluting vehicle without suffering from more than an amused conscience.

The reflection was cast upon Hahnemann that no one of his adherents could be found willing to act as his apothecary. Those who made this aspersion seem to have forgotten that in Germany apothecaries could only practice by special licence, and that only a certain number in ratio to the population were allowed.

Yet eventually from amongst the already licensed chemists Hahnemann was able to count upon followers. Amongst these were Apothecary Otto of Rotha, near Leipzig, and Apothecary Müller of Schöningen, near Brunswick, both men working at a little distance from large towns in which he had been resident. But it was Apothecary Lappe of Neudietendorf who was the first chemist who, from conviction, made himself familiar with Hahnemann's way of preparing medicines. A member of the Moravian community of Herrnhuters, he is described as an amiable old gentleman, not unlike Hahnemann in his manners, by a visitor who saw him sitting in a comfortable armchair with a long pipe in his mouth. This reminds us that Dr. Pfaff described Hahnemann as having the appearance of one belonging to the Herrnhuters or Moravians.

Another visitor, in *Sketches from the Notes of a Travelling Homœopath*, wrote:

> "The traveller wished to ascertain what kind of arrangement Herr Lappe had made. He found a part completely isolated from the general chemist's shop, which itself made a good impression from its extremely clean appearance. The traveller was able to convince himself that Herr Lappe was conscientiously following the homœopathic instructions, and affirms that the modest bearing of Herr Lappe himself convinced him of his accurate mode of procedure. The homœopathic medicines were made up and sold in small chests."

Here then, was the parent pharmacy of all the homœopathic pharmacies now existing.

Some suggestion was at this time made that Hahnemann should now resort to Prussian protection. He evidently also contemplated at one time the possibility of going to Altenburg. Both proposals fell through, but a letter to the ruling Duke of Anhalt-Köthen led to the issue of a Decree inviting Hahnemann to make his home in Köthen.

More than one reason was leading Hahnemann to expect a friendly attitude from this quarter. In the first place, Governor von Sternegg at the Court of Köthen had already been cured by Hahnemann's treatment, and, probably on Sternegg's advice, the Duke Ferdinand himself was Hahnemann's patient at the time of this correspondence. Further, the Duke was, like Hahnemann, a Freemason.

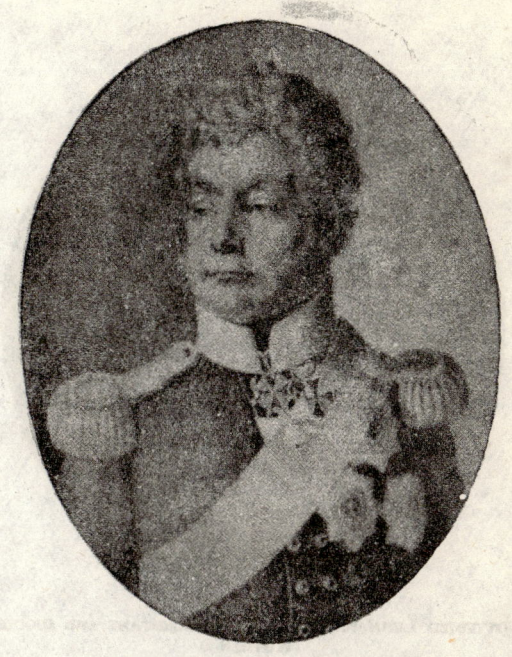

FERDINAND, DUKE OF ANHALT-KÖTHEN

Faces page 208

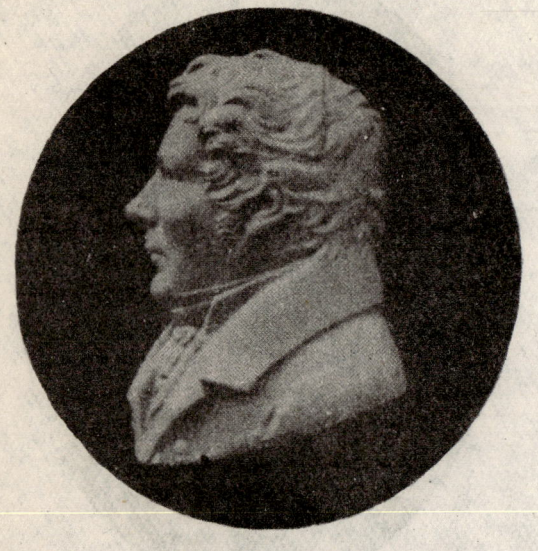

Dr. Gottfried Lehmann, Hahnemann's assistant and successor in Köthen

See page 221 *Faces page 209*

THE LEIPZIG APOTHECARIES

But, alas, in the wording of the ducal Decree, now received, the permission to dispense as well as prepare medicines was not included.

Bitterly disappointed on making this discovery, Hahnemann hastened, with the decree in hand, to his friend Adam Müller, the Austrian Consul-General in Saxony, who had already intervened on his behalf. Adam Müller describes the interview which followed:

> "I told him I had done everything I could in the matter; I could not possibly beg for another Decree from His Serene Highness. In my presence, and that of de Freygang and my son, the tears came into the eyes of this much insulted and irritated man; he declared confusedly that he could not speak in his usual way as his temper was irritable. I must confess that the sorrow of the man touched me deeply. I was convinced that before us sat one of the greatest physicians of the century, whose discoveries will only be appreciated in their full extent by posterity. I therefore promised to do all that was possible, and to forward my petition, so that His Serene Highness might notify me by a writ from the Cabinet. . . ."

Accordingly Müller, after considerable hesitation, wrote to Governor Sternegg in Köthen. He explained clearly that, had Dr. Hahnemann been willing only to prepare, without himself giving his medicines to his patients, there would have been no serious contention with the Leipzig

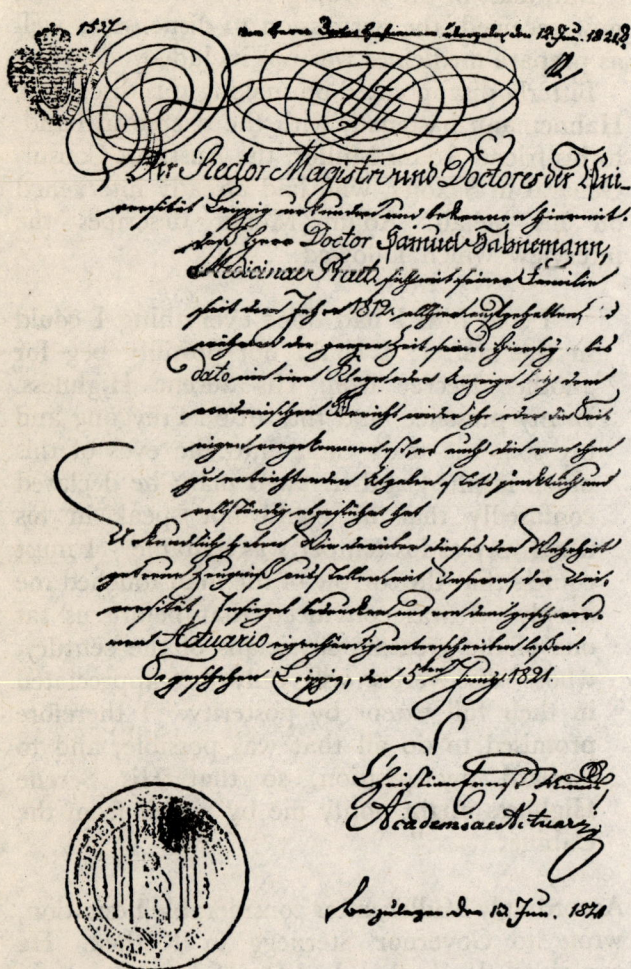

HAHNEMANN'S CERTIFICATE ON LEAVING LEIPZIG UNIVERSITY AT THE END OF NINE YEARS.

apothecaries, the necessary privilege for Hahnemann being that of self-dispensing.

The following personal reply from Prince Ferdinand himself, addressed from Köthen to Hahnemann and dated April 2nd, 1821, resulted:

"To Dr. Hahnemann of Leipzig.

"We reply to his request, that we willingly give him permission to establish himself in our town of residence, Köthen, as a practising physician. Also, in consideration of the fact that in our country all scientific research is given fair play, as an exception to the general rule, we wish to grant him the privilege of preparing with his own hands the remedies required for his treatments and of giving them to the patients under his care. Otherwise we remark that Dr. Hahnemann must submit himself to all other laws and police regulations of the country, and will therefore have to obey the directions of our Medical Council, from which, however, like all our subjects, he has the right of appeal to Us. We conclude with the desire for the happiest results in all the treatments of Dr. Hahnemann, so that his widespread reputation may increase and give us the opportunity of giving him proofs of our especial esteem and goodwill.

"Ferdinand, Duke of Anhalt."

The second person mentioned as present during Adam Müller's interview was Councillor de Freygang, Consul-General of Russia at Leipzig. Of him, the Swiss physician Dr. Peschier tells us that, after Hahnemann had left Leipzig, he sent twice a day over the eight leagues that divided the University city from Köthen to consult with Dr. Hahnemann at a time of acute illness in his household.

The Duke's letter sanctioning both the preparation and dispensing of medicines now made the prospect of going to Köthen entirely satisfactory. It bears, incidentally, the same date as the previous less satisfactory ducal Decree. It was as if the writer had wished it to be known that the fuller privilege had from the first been intended.

The practical sequel to these most happy communications was noticed in the *Korrespondent von und für Deutschland* of April 19th: "The inventor of the homœopathic system, Dr. Samuel Hahnemann, leaves Leipzig in the next few days, and will establish himself as a practising physician in Köthen." The article then announced the professional privileges that Hahnemann was to enjoy under the reigning Duke's protection, and proceeded:

"The Medical Council of Köthen has given by this act a praiseworthy example of real disinterestedness and of true regard to the progress of science. It was not thought justifiable to withhold shelter from this already ageing, true researcher, or to dispute the right of preparing and dispensing his own remedies with the most famous teacher of chemistry and pharmacy. To Dr. Hahnemann could not well be forbidden what he taught, seeing that for twenty years the apothecaries

THE LEIPZIG APOTHECARIES

of Germany have consulted his *Apotheker-Lexicon* in all cases of doubt. . . . A large number of patients, whose treatment was interrupted for several months on account of the persecution against Dr. Hahnemann which was going on in Leipzig, will now be able to follow their own inclinations unmolested and our free-thinking (!) country is spared the reproach of having suppressed one of the most remarkable discoveries for the welfare of humanity and of having purposely retarded one of the most comforting prospects for those who suffer."

The first part of Adam Müller's letter to Sternegg, already quoted in part, included the same reminder of the facts that Hahnemann was recognised as one of the most famous analytical and pharmaceutical chemists of Germany, and that most physicians and apothecaries had used his *Apotheker-Lexicon* as a guide for many years. We seem to trace the same pen at work in the Consul's letter and in the press announcement. Hahnemann did not get away from Leipzig until June of the year 1821.

CHAPTER XII

HAHNEMANN AS COURT PHYSICIAN

Köthen, 1821-1830

KÖTHEN, a quiet little town at the centre of a wide plain, is dominated by the two tall spires, with their curious connecting bridge, of the Protestant "Jakobskirche." It has long been shorn of its grand-ducal lustre, which was still there in Hahnemann's day; for years ago the Dukes removed their residence to Dessau, some 15 miles east, until the last of the race, together with his Dessau palace, was removed by the revolution of 1918.

Like every German town, large or small, Köthen is adorned by a number of sculptured monuments and statues, and amongst them is the Hahnemann "Denkmal," placed at crossroads under the shadow of a wooded public park. To the right of the Roman Goddess *Hygeia* stands a vigorous bust of Hahnemann, while on the left is one of Dr. Lutze, his medical successor in Köthen, who lived long in the house opposite the memorial, where his son and two of his grandsons, all homœopathic physicians, still reside and practise.

Stephen Hobhouse, a visitor in 1931 to the home of Dr. Lutze, wrote:

"I was warmly entertained by these three. On the staircase is a coloured glass window showing the portraits of Hahnemann and Lutze with botanical emblems, notably digitalis and aconite, and Æsculapius' serpent. I was then taken to Wall-strasse, where Hahnemann on leaving Leipzig settled down, then a more open and dignified street than it is to-day. His house forms one side of an obtuse angle, and seen from the garden is quite picturesque because of its large covered wooden balcony running round the angle of the house. Immediately behind is a small paved court, then the garden itself, about 40 by 8 yards in size, whilst beyond are the remains of the old town wall—hence the name of Wall-strasse. A temporary shelter covered with scarlet runners is the only reminder of Hahnemann's summer-house, long since removed, where he used to sit and work."

It can be readily imagined with what peculiar satisfaction Hahnemann, now *Hofrat* or Court Physician, took up his abode in this modest corner house in Köthen, a free physician able to pursue his profession according to his deepest convictions born of a wide and varied experience. He lived, however, at first at the "Grand Hostelry," for his future house required some adaptations.

With a hall large enough for a living room and a roomy upper landing, the rest of the rooms of 270 Wall Street (later No. 47) were small. The entrance hall was used partly as a waiting room for patients, whilst running from it to the left was the consulting room. One of the frequent friendly visitors here was Principal Albrecht of the Seminary in Köthen, who had known Hahnemann from the days when he used to sing short lullabies to his children, and write little poems for them "in the most affable and fatherly way." It is he who has confirmed the impression left by the memoirs of Franz Hartmann, the medical student, and Ernst von Brunnow, the young lawyer, that Hahnemann felt happiest among his family and showed here better than anywhere else his amiable, happy, and cheerful disposition.

Home life, indeed, always lay happily at the back of his multitudinous responsibilities and concerns. Principal Albrecht describes this with even more detail than Dr. Lutze, who visited him in Köthen. Wall-strasse, he tells us, was the widest and most beautiful street in the town at the time. To the right of the great oak door in Hahnemann's house were three large windows with dark green shutters, whilst on the other side there were two. The roomy hall was lighted by a large staircase window, and to its right was the sitting room where his friends assembled. Opposite was the doctor's consultation room and study. Miniatures of his daughters, by Schoppe of Berlin, hung on the chief wall; there was also a portrait of himself by the same painter, and a portrait bust modelled by Steinhaüser. By the window stood the old-fashioned grand piano ("old-fashioned" to a contemporary, it must be noted) round which Hahnemann liked to sit in the circle of his family.

On the mantelpiece of this, Hahnemann's sanctum, were several clocks for which he had a special liking, winding them daily himself. The doctor burnt in his room only a tallow light, of which he often made use to light his pipe. Yet the garden, it seems, was Hahnemann's favourite retreat, and the little bower at the end saw not only literary work accomplished under the shade of its ivy, but was also the place chosen sometimes for breakfast, and even on occasions patients consulted him there. In its seclusion, moreover, the sculptor Steinhauser made his bust of the doctor.

Perhaps, too, it was amongst its ivy leaves that he observed the industrious spider at her web-building and on her travels. Writing to Dr. Stapf in 1827, he says:

"The books on entomology are excellent. I thank you for sending them to me. But they do not solve the riddle respecting spiders. To judge from my own experiments, they appear to possess a power still unknown to us to project themselves forward in the air—not on shot-out threads. In my experiments I made this impossible, and I saw one, suspended by its thread from my finger, first hover in the air in a horizontal position, then dart obliquely upwards, where it disappeared from my sight."

Here in his garden it was that he walked to and fro with one or another of his daughters under the stars sometimes till midnight in summer or, if the stars were obscured, with a lantern in hand, thus easing heart and mind of its burdens before requiring of sleep its respite. The medical student Hornburg also speaks of patrolling the garden with him by the light of a swinging lamp. Sometimes the companion was a little dog who also sat very close to the doctor at meals.

After only a few months' residence (as it appears from a letter of the Austrian Consul in Leipzig to Friedrich von Gentz, one of the German political writers who openly and violently attacked Napoleon) Hahnemann had the triumph in Köthen of completely curing an inflammation of the lungs without venesection by homœopathic minimal doses, a cure which so far had been regarded as an impossibility.

But there was to be a still more obvious tribute to the doctor's powers. In the press, in March of 1824, announcement was made that the Duke, who had been suffering from a dangerous nerve affection, was now out of danger, thanks to the efforts of Hahnemann.

Some weeks later a pronouncement from the Duke himself, dated April 28th, sanctioned the appointment of Dr. Mossdorf as an assistant to Hahnemann. It read thus:

"To our High State Government.
"I have decided, so that the lower ranks of my domestics may be no longer kept from the benefits of homœopathic treatment, to pay Dr. Mossdorf the annual sum of 60 Florins, to treat and provide gratuitously with medicine all those domestics who have hitherto received free medicine, and who now wish to avail

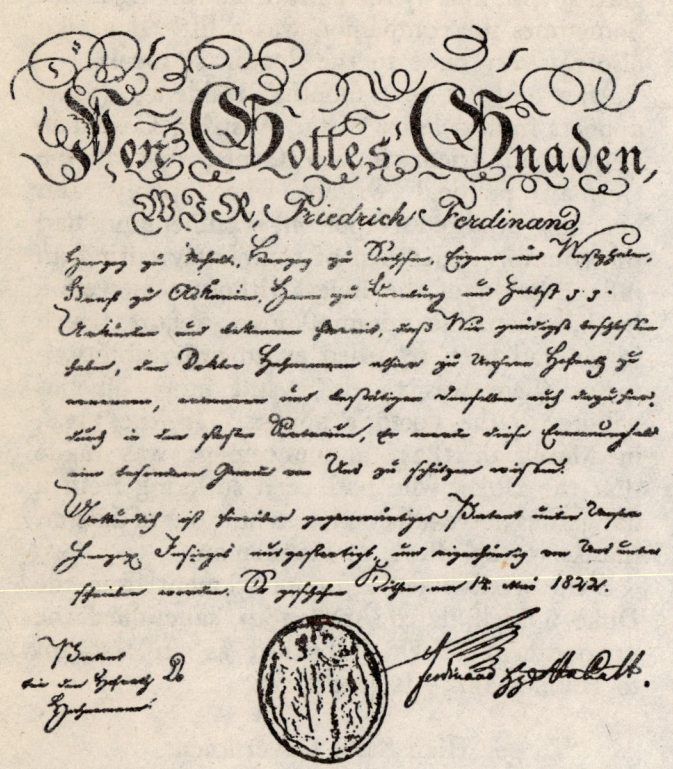

DUCAL PATENT APPOINTING HAHNEMANN AS *Hofrat*.

themselves of his help and the homœopathic method of treatment.

"Ferdinand."

The marriage of one of Hahnemann's daughters to this doctor unfortunately brought the sorrow of an unhappy alliance into the family circle. Later the post of Assistant Physician was given to Dr. Lehmann, who proved an invaluable colleague and life-long friend.

Rather more than a year later Hahnemann received a letter from the Duchess of Anhalt couched in almost affectionate terms:

"It would be impossible, my dearest Hofrat, for me to start on such a long journey as I have before me, without expressing to you my thanks for all the sympathy which you showed me. Rest assured that my heart remembers such debts. Your treatment of myself I always consider only as interrupted. I hope that on my return you may find a more receptive soil for your remedies. Please be so good as to give me a few words regarding the state of health of the Duke, and remember

"Julie, Duchess of Anhalt."

From a letter addressed to the Royal Prussian Consul-General, Dr. Baumgärtner, by Hahnemann in 1823, we find that the doctor was in no sense resting on his laurels as Court Physician. In this he writes: "I regard it as the work of Divine Providence that you, a man of high standing in the world, should have the foresight and courage to try and bring honour to the new art of healing, which has been maligned in a thousand ways." Hahnemann then describes his long search for the keystone to the cure of chronic diseases, and his belief that he has seen light upon the matter. "This knowledge," he continues, "now finally attained, is of such a kind that I could impart it to young physicians in a practical way, at the bedside of patients, in some clinical establishment through their own observations." He then states that he had already confided his wish for hospital opportunities to the reigning Duke Ferdinand of Anhalt-Köthen. At the same time he indicates that, despite the Duke's cordial sympathy, it was unlikely that anything would be done, since in Köthen there was no hospital in existence. We can readily imagine the opposition from the medical authorities with which any endeavour on the part of the Duke to open a hospital with a view to offering facilities to Hahnemann would have been met. Time indeed proved Hahnemann's hopes in this direction to be vain.

It was in this year that Dr. Karl Aegidi came as a patient into Hahnemann's hands. For two years, since being thrown from his carriage in 1820, this physician had suffered so much that he had to abandon his profession and entrust himself entirely to the care of his colleagues. Every remedy of the orthodox school had been tried, and at length Dr. Aegidi in January, 1823, wrote to Hahnemann telling him exactly what had been done. In reply a letter was received scathing in its condemnation of the "issues," "setons," and, finally, the chief torture, "cautery," which had been used. Hahnemann wrote, too, that he suspected some previous infection. Dr. Aegidi then remembered that after pricking himself with a needle when performing a small operation, his arm had once swollen, leaving pain in the left shoulder. "Now," he wrote, "I could look at the reason for my disease in quite another light," and taking the treatment Hahnemann prescribed, the end of about six weeks he awoke to a sense of health all the sweeter for his having been so long a stranger to it. Hahnemann, whom he visited in Köthen, continued the treatment, "after which," wrote Aegidi, "my illness disappeared entirely."

After a close study of the principles of homœopathy, we find Dr. Aegidi choosing the new method with his patients, and later still becoming the founder, with the Countess von der Recke, of the first Homœopathic Hospital for Children, which was in Düsselthal.

We can now picture Hahnemann at work on what proved to be his last medical book of importance, entitled *Chronic Diseases, Their Nature and Homœopathic Treatment*. Those of his opponents who wished to belittle the doctor's judgment sought to do so now by levelling the absurd criticism that Hahnemann in this work had confused what he described as the latent nameless taint in the system which hindered the cure of chronic disorders with the specific complaint, the itch. This was because for the broader predisposition to disease Hahnemann used the word

Psora. We know, however, that from the time of Celsus (30 A.D.) to Willan (1798) it was far more widely applied than to the skin disease caused by the itch-parasite. Here was but another instance of a willingness to be excused from investigating the deeper implications of the doctor's teaching. That there was no confusion in Hahnemann's mind is evidenced by the fact that for the two types of ailment—the particular psora or "itch" and the general "psora"—his prescriptions were diametrically opposed.

To Hahnemann psora was a disease or disposition to disease, hereditary from generation to generation for thousands of years. "The hermit on Montserrat in his rocky abode can escape it as little as the young prince in his cambric swaddling clothes." No wonder, pondering deeply on this, he bent all his mind to the discovery of some reliable counteraction to this disastrous inherent tendency. "Lo!", he wrote, "in this time the Giver of all good things suffered me to solve this sublime riddle for mankind's good as a result of incessant thought, tireless investigation, accurate observation, and the most careful experiments."

Despite a considerable measure of alienation amongst his own followers produced by the appearance of Hahnemann's last literary work, owing to certain exaggerations in it from which he afterwards withdrew without altering the main thesis, friendly relations with them seem to have been re-established completely by the following year. On August 10th, 1829, the Doctor's jubilee, commemorating the fiftieth

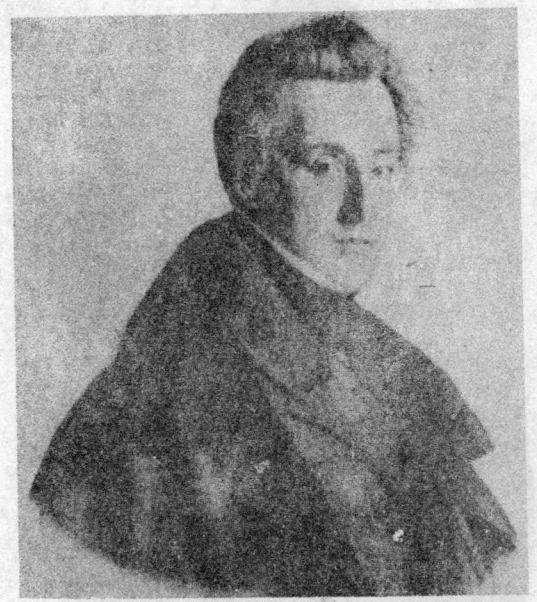

MEDIZINALRAT DR. K. J. AEGIDI, FOUNDER OF THE FIRST HOMŒOPATHIC HOSPITAL FOR CHILDREN.

See page 222 *Faces page 224*

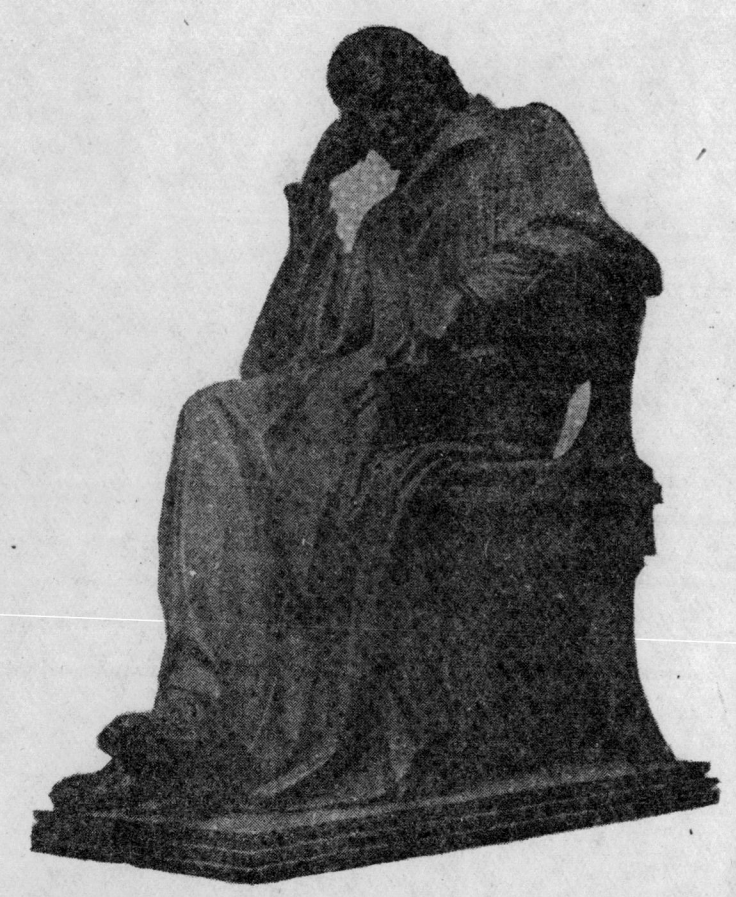

CENTRAL FIGURE OF THE HAHNEMANN MEMORIAL IN WASHINGTON, U.S.A.

See page 250 *Faces page 225*

year since his qualification at Erlangen, was celebrated.

While planning the festal jubilee, his friends desired to obtain a reliable portrait and medal to present to him for the occasion, and some difficulty was experienced in getting Hahnemann to sit without suspecting the intention. These difficulties Dr. Rummel managed to overcome. In the correspondence we note Hahnemann's unwillingness to sit for an inferior painter. In one of his letters to Rummel we read:

> "I am not as vain as Alexander, the conqueror of the world, *qui nec pingi, nisi ab Apelle, nec fingi volebat, nisi a Praxitele*, but I have no desire to see another copy made of the unsuccessful oil painting. . . . Should I live, and should some good portrait-painter come in my way, I would get my likeness taken, and that in a larger size than the last as you desire. But should this not happen, then let us leave things as they are, let me only be handed down to posterity in the spiritual features of the inner man which are not indistinctly portrayed in what I have written. My vanity does not go beyond this."

Yet once the object of his friends was obtained we can imagine that Hahnemann was a willing victim, for contact with artists was no doubt a refreshment to a man of his temperament. The result was that during the spring and summer of that year Hahnemann was additionally preoccupied. Whilst continuing to work on the *Materia Medica* and keeping up his wide correspondence in addition to his practice and visitors, considerable time was given to sittings for his two artists, the young sculptor, Dietrich, and Schoppe, the portrait painter. Such was the pressure on him, in a letter to Stapf he says: "I never read the *Allgemeine Anzeiger*, because I have no time to do so. Even the political papers lie by me for days before I can look at them. My time is much taken up, months fly past like days."

When the day of the doctor's Jubilee arrived, nothing was lacking to spread abroad an atmosphere of personal affection and public gratitude. Baron von Gersdorff, after his address of congratulation, presented a document written in Latin signed by all present, about 500 persons from every European country. Dr. Mühlebein presented him with 1250 thalers to form the beginning of a fund for a homœopathic clinic. From the Medical Faculty at Erlangen University came a diploma and congratulations. Dr. Stapf, his intimate friend as well as colleague, presented the doctor with an edition of his own *Lesser Writings*, published in collected form for the first time.

The Duke and Duchess of Anhalt-Köthen both made presentations. The Duke wrote:

> "You have done such great and lasting service to mankind by discovering and establishing the system of homœopathy, which now is already spreading over all parts of the world, that I gladly include myself among the numbers of those admirers who have assembled

this day to bring you the tribute of their gratitude."

A letter from the Duchess struck the same note:

"You have now reached a wonderful point from which you can look back upon a long lapse of years spent in useful activity. In the wide diffusion of homœopathy you can see the most beautiful fruit of your many endeavours now ripening for the welfare of humanity."

By far the most important outcome of this was the formation of a Society of Homœopathic Physicians to meet annually on the same date. The first meeting was held in Leipzig the year following. Subsequently this body undertook the founding of the proposed homœopathic clinic in Leipzig—a hospital which, alas, brought considerable sorrow to Hahnemann. This was incidentally due to the appearance amongst his followers of what he termed the "half-homœopaths." It was obviously imperative that only pure homœopathy should be practised in an institution founded to illustrate to the world its more beneficial methods. But its founder's intolerance of those medical men who desired to use the methods of both schools in alternation was extreme; so clearly contrasted were the issues in his own mind, and so jealous was he in these later years of this isolated opportunity for a clear corporate demonstration of his new science and art for the healing of his fellows.

Eight days after the Jubilee Hahnemann wrote to Dr. Stapf:

"Dear Colleague, I can bear much joy and sorrow, but I was hardly able to stand the surprise of so many and such strong proofs of the kindness and affection of my pupils and friends. . . . Now that I gradually regain my mental equilibrium and ponderingly examine each present which was given to me with such kindness of heart I wonder more and more! . . . I have not deserved it. These are gifts of generosity, delicacy and excessive gratitude, whose value I fully appreciate. . . . I beg of you kindly to communicate these feeble utterances of mine to those concerned and to keep a large portion for yourself. . . . Convey my cordial greetings and appreciation to my friends Rummel, Gross, Franz and Gerstoff."

A second letter to the same, over a month later, begins:

"You have rendered an immense service to me by your appropriately arranged collection and publication of my *Lesser Writings*. . . . It is only within the last few days, owing to an accumulation of work, that I have been able properly to look through your kind, well-planned and well-executed undertaking. I do not know how I am still to get through such a quantity of work. But what we do so willingly, only fatigues us till bedtime; and in the morning, thank God, there is a complete return to strength. I must close to-day with kindest regards from my family to you, your wife and family and also from me. Your friend, S. Hahnemann."

This ending, including as it does greetings from and to all the family on both sides, is eminently characteristic of Hahnemann's sense of family wholeness. The volume of *Lesser Writings* in its English translation has unfortunately been long out of print. It is to be hoped that at least a judicious selection of its attractive and interesting essays will be republished.

Amongst the greetings received at the celebration of the medical Jubilee was one from Constantine Hering, expressing his joy at having been able to carry the good seed of the Doctor's teaching as far as America. This man as a medical student had attended Hahnemann's lectures in Leipzig, but became especially attached in his work to Dr. Robbi who, like Clarus, was an active antagonist to homœopathy. The publisher Baumgartner had in those days approached Dr. Robbi, with a view to obtaining from him a book against the new medical science. Being too pressed with work, Robbi suggested that Constantine Hering, his youthful assistant, should do it instead. In order to make his shafts more effective, the young man both studied the works of Hahnemann and became involved in some "provings." The results of his experiments were such that before long the medical student became convinced of the truth of homœopathy.

At one time it appears that Constantine Hering's instructor, Dr. Robbi, had approached Hahnemann in a letter with a view to possibly becoming a follower of the new method. In Hahnemann's long reply to Robbi we find nothing but considerations calculated to discourage a man in whom apparently he had little or no faith. If we compare this with a letter addressed to Constantine Hering soon after his avowal of homœopathy, we can trace more precisely his mistrust of the tutor and the complete confidence which he clearly placed in the younger man, to whom he wrote thus:

". . . As you wish to procure a Doctor's degree in the old system of medicine next spring, I beg and counsel you not to allow your homœopathic opinions to be known by the allopathic physicians of Leipzig, least of all by that most implacable of all allopaths, Clarus, if you do not wish to be grievously tormented at your examination or even rejected. . . . Yet, when you have got your degree and have pitched upon the place of your future practice, then fear nothing more from the obstacles which the Corporation of Apothecaries will be able to put in your way. Some escape will open by which you will be able to put the good method into practice.

"I have confidence in you and am not afraid of being wrong in regarding you as one of the few of my followers who will practise the divine art among your afflicted fellow men under the eye of the All-present. Then, while you will not miss obtaining the so-called temporal gain, you will also secure the approval of your conscience without which kingdoms cannot give happiness. . . . Only he who is good can be sure of the support of God, without whom we can accomplish nothing, from whom everything comes which contributes to the cure of His beloved family of man.

"Of your offer to make experiments with medicines upon yourself, with the help of your sister, I will make use when you are in a place and position to practise your art."

Constantine Hering, we know, did not conceal his changed opinion from the Leipzig professors, but in consequence was led to obtain his degree in Würzburg. Hering's adoption of homœopathy had subsequently the far-reaching effect of converting Baumgärtner, the Leipzig publisher, at whose request the attack on homœopathy was to have been written. As a result Baumgärtner not only became the publisher of one of Hahnemann's most uncompromising pamphlets, but later he promoted the journal *Allgemeine Homœopathische Zeitung*, which Dr. Rummel edited for twenty-two years.

From the Court of Weimar a request for the doctor's advice came from the Countess von Pappenheim, to whom two daughters had been born as the mistress of Jerome Napoleon, brother to the Emperor Napoleon, who had made him King of Westphalia. At the time of her appeal to Hahnemann for his assistance, Jenny, one of these two daughters, was still unaware of her parentage on the father's side. Though later this was revealed to her by her sister, before the latter entered a convent; and Jenny and her father, Jerome Napoleon, afterwards corresponded affectionately for several years. The occasion of the trouble was that Jenny, now at the age of sixteen, had fallen deeply in love with a young Englishman, who afterwards succumbed to consumption. They were therefore obliged to abandon all further thought of marriage, and her lover left her. An illness resulted.

Lily Braun, a descendant of Jenny Pappenheim, in her book *In the Shadow of the Titans*, tells us that, as none of the physicians in Weimar could help Jenny, her mother turned to Dr. Hahnemann, whose reputation, we know from Hufeland and Goethe, had already reached that town. With Goethe, now an old man, Jenny and her mother were personally acquainted. A correspondence covering over a year ensued between the doctor and his youthful patient—youthful, yet already mature in thought and feeling, and living in a resplendent Court not without its vein of corruption.

Several extracts from Hahnemann's letters will serve as a mirror in which we may trace something of the features of both the writer and the recipient. The first is dated November, 1827:

> "Your unhappy thoughts are only effects of your bodily ailments, which in your case must have begun as far back as early childhood. But, as your body recovers health,

these depressing ideas will disappear altogether. Still, I consider that this melancholy disposition has up to the present been of the greatest advantage to your moral nature. It has preserved you from the levity which so often prevents young ladies of your age from pursuing the high ideals for which they were created and makes them a sacrifice to a frivolity which is fashionable. Thus, an all-loving Providence has through this spiritual suffering shown His care over you in the safeguarding of your noble nature. For the purity of that nature is worth more than all the riches of the East."

In the following spring Hahnemann again wrote to Jenny:

"In your maturer years, at any rate, when your heart will be stronger and beat more calmly and your internal ailments are still nearer cure, there are many happier, serener days before you. The feelings, difficult to name, which still assail you now, will then be easily dispersed in a restful, joyous life and in the happy marriage which you deserve, with the lovely duties of wifehood and motherhood. Only be comforted! The nobility of your mind will help to bring things right before long. For I perceive you do not make too large claims upon this somewhat imperfect world, and are working out more your own perfection."

Our last extract is from one of the letters concluding the correspondence:

"Please continue, while attending as you do to my advice on diet, to reveal to me in your letters the state of your mind, as well as of your heart and feelings. You have to do with an old man who is unusually receptive of such information, and who takes a most sincere interest in it, yes, and who knows too how to give you good advice in such matters. In a case like yours, when the mental factor and sensitiveness of soul get the upper hand, the bodily factor is held in subjection and becomes excessively disturbed. So it becomes necessary to guide both back into the right way of life in which body as well as mind may claim its rights, and the imagination, moreover, may be as little as possible excited, while the powers of thinking and observation are exercised. For the present I beg you to read only light, cheerful lyrics (no other poetry), well-written and truthful books of travel, biographies and history. And, so as to give you on your walks a much greater sense of pleasure, you have, living in Weimar, the best opportunity to secure a tutor who is no pedant; and he, in the company of your respected mother, will impart to you knowledge which will in the future be much more welcome and valuable to you than many other feminine occupations."

Hahnemann was no doubt here again thinking, amongst other things, of botany.

About a year after the celebrations for

Hahnemann's doctorate, the importance and weight of work yielded to the pressure of a personal event in the house in Wall-strasse. This was the death of Henriette, his wife. Essentially a German "Hausfrau," homely and practical in the extreme, nevertheless Hahnemann was able to speak of her as "the noble companion of his professional life."

Principal Albrecht also has appreciatively sketched for us this remarkably strong personality. He writes that she was "a capable woman of energetic character, of unusually high culture for these days, and of great personal kindness." Yet Ernst von Brunnow disliked Frau Hahnemann, describing her as "the scolding Xanthippe," who gave her husband "many a bitter hour, and exercised a most baneful influence on him." Franz Hartmann, on the other hand, whilst admitting that she ruled her husband and no doubt the household, adds, "yet he let it willingly happen, in the belief that he owed this tribute to his wife, as she watched over all his peculiarities with the greatest attention and punctuality." Albrecht comments on the fact that she had considerable musical faculty, setting her own poems sometimes to music. Further, we are told that Henriette Hahnemann had sacrificed to her husband the whole of her moderate property at the time when he formed the resolution to withdraw from practice to seek better methods whereby to relieve the sufferings of his fellow men. Nor is there any doubt that she watched with tender care over his domestic happiness and well-being, "so that he only felt happy in his home and in his family, and seldom left them," a responsibility in which his daughters had long shared and which now, after the death of their mother, fell entirely to them.

There is evidence that in this respect the daughters were not lacking either in capacity or will. We have already noted that they also were concerned in helping their father with his work, preparing medicines, and sharing in the "provings," besides in such small attentions as relighting his pipe, if it should go out, and, more especially, refreshing him with music.

CHAPTER XIII

INTERNATIONAL DEVELOPMENTS

Köthen, 1830-1832

ANOTHER of Hahnemann's guests, Dr. Griesselich, tells us that at this time the doctor showed no traces of declining strength, despite the expenditure of a prodigious amount of energy. Whilst his white locks, emerging from beneath the velvet cap which covered his bald crown, hinted at his years, the impression left was otherwise of a sturdy figure.

"Hahnemann," wrote Griesselich, "is lively and brisk; every movement is full of life. His eyes reveal his inquiring spirit; they flash with the fire of youth. . . . His language is fiery and fluent; often it becomes vehement as a stream of lava against the enemies and opponents, not of himself personally, for to that he never alludes, but of the great truths to the testing of which he has summoned his colleagues for many decades."

The period from 1829 to 1832 Rapou, the French physician who had been with Hahnemann in Köthen, records as three very happy years in Hahnemann's experience, "honoured by the friendship and protection of a generous Prince, glorying in a reputation more than European, chief of a school whose pupils were zealous and respected. His practice was very large." This physician from Lyons in a letter describing his own visit to what he calls "the Mecca of Homœopathy," after speaking of the seemingly long hours spent in waiting for the dismissal of the patients and of the cordiality of the welcome he received on being admitted to the doctor's room, continues:

"Time passed rapidly and already we were conversing as two friends. I told him how I had learned of his new system, and of my success in its practical application; and he explained to me his opinions on the chronicity of diseases, on the method of their attack and the difficulty in curing them, also that certain so-called incurable affections ought not to be so regarded by the homœopath. . . . This long and interesting conversation was prolonged during a supper amicably offered and sumptuously served by the two daughters of Hahnemann, who rivalled each other in politeness and attention to their respected father. . . . At the hotel where I was staying it was customary to hear many times during the day the tramping of horses on the arrival and departure of the strangers who attended from all parts on account of the great reputation and successful practice of Hahnemann. This hotel at the time had a majority of its chambers occupied by persons who had come from distances to consult the oracle of Homœopathy; for example, I noticed among others a Dane, a Courlander, a Hungarian, a Russian and a Silesian."

Peschier, a French doctor from Geneva, who was numbered amongst these visitors, tells how at the end of the arduous day he found the doctor occupied in consultation on an infant, the child of a poor mother, upon whom he bestowed unwearied attentions. To this is added the significant observation, "for the poor were the same to him as those who had riches." Indeed, it was the exhaustive care spent on this single case that most impressed the French visitor, and led him to study the method further and to leave us his impressions.

Amongst others who went to Köthen was the Counsellor de Freygang, Consul-General of Russia at Leipzig. "His respect for Hahnemann," says Peschier, who was there at the same time, "is without limit, and it is, they say, to his zeal and affection that the latter owes the protection of the Duke of Anhalt."

When the above letter was reproduced by Bradford the documents since unearthed by Dr. Richard Haehl from the State archives of the ducal family at Zerbst had not yet been discovered. We now know that although de Freygang was present at the dramatic interview between Hahnemann and Adam Müller, the Austrian Consul-General in Saxony, concerning the freedom both to prepare and to dispense his own remedies, it was to the latter that Hahnemann chiefly owed an active intervention.

It is clear, however, that both the Austrian and Russian consuls were his convinced supporters, both before and after his leaving Leipzig.

We must not be deceived into thinking of the Köthen years as an era of peaceful retreat in the midst of strenuous but congenial occupations. To think of them as a time of undisturbed happiness would be, as Haehl warns us, a serious mistake.

> "More and more violent attacks on him and on his system succeeded one another continuously. But Hahnemann, like the general officer commanding in a battle, was hidden away behind the front and usually did nothing but supply the lines of direction for the answering thrust."

The carrying out of the plans was left to disciples, mostly his early pupils and friends, Dr. Stapf in Naumburg and Dr. Gross in Jüterbogk. The former, indeed, became "his dearest confidant and brother-in-arms, to whom he had recourse in all controversies and attacks and also in professional contingencies."

We can now turn out of the way a little to watch the activity of another of Hahnemann's followers, Dr. Aegidi, after his appointment to the Princess Friedrich of Prussia (who was already a homœopath) in Düsseldorf.

From that city Dr. Aegidi wrote that he had succeeded in winning the Prince her husband's interest and that he now had become his patient. In a further letter in the same month, Dr. Aegidi states:

"I think that they mean to accomplish nothing less than the return of the Princess to allopathic hands, but they need time for that, as, on account of her decided character, they cannot possibly precipitate matters with her. The consideration which people in high authority have to take of their subordinates goes so far, that the Prince recommended me to prescribe secretly. They prefer to put the Prince's son, Alexander [who had been subject to nervous attacks from early childhood] under Dr. Prieger of Kreutznach, who applied against these dynamic disturbances of the nervous system the moxa on the delicate spine of the eleven year old child every eight days— and proposes, if this experiment [!] should have no result, even to trephine [!!!]; sooner than trust him to a cautious homœopathic treatment, from which no damaging consequences are to be feared, but only good results might be expected—for the sole reason that the Governor of the Prince thinks nothing of homœopathy and does not wish to do so."*

The above letter was dated in September, 1831. In one which follows two months later, written, one imagines, with a sigh of deep relief, a marginal note is to be found: "The Prince has now appointed me physician to his two sons; I have now the whole family." The November letter ends with the comment: "The cholera greatly stimulates the liking for homœopathy."

* The "moxa" was a cylinder of readily combustible material, which is burnt on the skin; to "trephine" is to remove a part of the bone of the skull.

This brings us to the sudden and widespread publicity into which a single prescription of Hahnemann's was brought. This prescription, camphor, was directed to the arresting of the tragic epidemic of Asiatic cholera which was travelling rapidly, and with a heavy death-toll, from one country of Europe to another, during 1831 to 1832. One of Hahnemann's pamphlets dealing with this question, through the influence of the Anhalt doctors, was suppressed by the less favourable Duke Heinrich who had succeeded his brother Ferdinand in 1830. Several essays on *Cure of Cholera* followed one another and remarkable results attended the taking of Hahnemann's advice. As he had not treated or even seen one single cholera patient, the important question arose as to how Hahnemann had found his remedy with such complete conviction, and been able to make helpful suggestions with such confidence. The answer lay in the fact that Hahnemann had procured a very accurate description of the symptoms and had found that the first and most important of these in cholera patients resembled one another, and were similar to the symptoms produced if camphor was taken in large quantities by a healthy individual. Hahnemann had therefore concluded from the great similarity of the symptoms at the beginning of the disease with those brought out by camphor in the provings, that this ought to be the best remedy to give at the outset. In a like way he also prescribed the other remedies required for the cure of the later stages of cholera.

Anticipating the findings of the researches of such men as Pasteur and Koch, Hahnemann in his work on "the Mode and Propagation of Cholera," wrote:

> "The most striking infections took place and made astonishing progress . . . whenever . . . . the cholera miasm found an element favourable to its own multiplication and throve to an enormously increased swarm of those infinitely small, invisible living organisms, which are so murderously hostile to human life and which most probably form the infectious matter of cholera."

Whilst Hufeland held that cholera was of an "epidemically atmospheric, telluric nature," and spread abroad only through the air, Hahnemann, attributing it to a diminutive organism of a lower nature, maintained that it was capable of propagation by personal contact. This led him to demand urgently isolation and disinfection, and to make the statement that the physicians and nurses were the most certain and frequent propagators of the contagion. Keen, too, were his thrusts at the former for their methods.

> "They seem to prefer," he wrote, "delivering over all mankind to the grave-digger, to listening to the good counsel of the new, purified healing art; but who can prevent them acting so, as they alone possess the power in the State to suppress what is good?"

These were, no doubt, the passages the deletion of which had been demanded of Hahnemann by the authorities in Köthen. Of such import were they to him, however, that he accepted the ban of censorship on the essay in which they appeared in that town (although he was Court Physician there) rather than omit them. It was afterwards published in Leipzig, but the sale was still prohibited in Köthen. No one who has not witnessed the reckless propagation of such a calamitous scourge, through ignorance or indifference to rational precautions, can quite grasp the purport of such vehemence.

An increasing number of enquirers from all over Germany and beyond now got into touch with the doctor in Köthen. Amongst these was the Medical Officer of Health, Beumelburg, of Pruss in Holland, one of eight physicians appointed by the ruling monarch to meet the ravages of the epidemic. From the Municipal Sanitary Commission of the Province of Warmsdoff also came a request for the remedy. It was written from Gösten and dated October 23rd, 1831.

> "Very esteemed Hofrat,
> "You were so good as to supply the capital, Köthen, with the prophylactic for cholera, free of charge, and Master-mason Busse, who has seen you, says you are willing to do the same for us, if we request you to do so. We should not like to miss the opportunity of making use of this patriotic offer, and request of you, Sir, the remedies required for this town. . . . We recognise your kindness with deep gratitude and are glad of the opportunity to assure you of our deep esteem."

From Brünn in Moravia, from Lemberg, from Wischnei-Woltschek, from Daka, and elsewhere reports of good results were also forthcoming. Dr. Bakody, whose remarkable figures of cure under homœopathy were doubted by the authorities in Raab, was able to produce 112 accredited testimonies of cure out of the 148 cured, the signatures including a Councillor of the Consistory, a High Advocate, and several ministers. Dr. Lövy of Prague, writing to Hahnemann about a visit he had paid to Vienna, stated: "Homœopathy acts wonderfully in cholera." From this doctor Hahnemann also received a request to get into touch with a Father Veith in Vienna, a priest of the Ligurian order with a medical degree, now a preacher at the Cathedral of St. Stephen. In Austria Hahnemann's new method of treatment was still prohibited by an Imperial Mandate, but Father Veith did not hesitate to show his convictions openly. With the Austrian nobility and the officials of the Court before him in the Cathedral he went so far when preaching as to extol the blessings belonging to the homœopathic treatment, adding the observation that, in his judgment, it was no insignificant indication when in the same part of the earth which was the birthplace of cholera the powerful remedy camphor was to be found indigenous. In point of fact this flagrant setting aside of the Imperial Mandate was no startling event. Already countless persons in various stations of life in Vienna were known to be ignoring it and using the prescription of Hahnemann's recommendation. In reply to the communications from Father Veith, Hahnemann wrote with warm appreciation, picturing vividly it may be the scene of this priest's activities, since his own training had been partly in the Austrian capital. From Prague Dr. Anton Schmidt, Physician-in-Ordinary to the Duchess of Lucca, wrote to Köthen:

> "In Vienna they insist very emphatically that cholera is epidemic and not contagious; the peasants in the surrounding villages take no notice of this view, they threaten to kill every Viennese who dares to come to a village. . . . That your little book is read, though secretly, is very certain."

From this it transpires that many were still careful lest their use of Hahnemann's beneficent prescription should be detected. As the transmission of the cholera germ through contaminated water supplies had not yet been discovered, even by the authorities, the ignorance of the peasantry with its touch of tragic terror is not to be wondered at.

In November, 1831, Hahnemann confided to Dr. Stapf that he had received from several Prussian cities requests to procure for them a capable homœopathic physician, adding characteristically: "I shall do that very willingly and irrespective of trouble and small expenses, but they must choose a fearless and reliable man with whom I could exchange letters on the subject." We read also of a young doctor appointed as homœopathic family physician to an English family resident in Nice.

In August, 1831, we find Hahnemann writing to Dr. Schweikert of a post in England:

"Dear friend and colleague,
"The first Earl by rank in England, Lord Shrewsbury, a very religious Catholic peer, who lives on his estate (like a great prince) asks me to provide him with a good homœopathic physician. He brought from Naples to his English estate a few years ago the famous homœopath, Dr. Romani, who caused a great sensation there with his cures, and even in London. But the colder climate did not suit him. The Earl then fetched another Italian homœopath (for my Lord and his whole family cling body and soul to homœopathy) from Fabiano, Rabata by name, but he can no longer keep his post as family physician on account of some caries of the clavicle, the result of an old shot wound. He is going to London for treatment and will then return to his family in Italy. . . . The daughters and their governess, who is German, speak German perfectly; the married daughter, Countess Talbot, with whom I had some small professional dealings last year, writes a very good German letter, so that it would be very useful for you to have such social intercourse. . . . I am therefore waiting for your considered decision. . . ."

Yet another convert to Hahnemann's methods was found in the English physician Dr. F. F.

Quin. Quin, who is styled as "the last of the English wits," was appointed physician to Napoleon I. But the great Emperor died before Dr. Quin's appointment had taken effect. Subsequently he was made family physician in England to Prince Leopold of Saxe-Coburg, later King of the Belgians, and uncle to Queen Victoria.

It was in Naples that Dr. Quin had met Dr. Necker, a disciple of Hahnemann's. This had led him to visit Leipzig in order to meet the founder of the new system of therapeutics as far back as 1826.

During the epidemic of cholera on the Continent, Dr. Quin went to Moravia to study that disease, and as the result of a deeper insight into the effective workings of Hahnemann's method was led on his return to practice homœopathy first in King Street, St. James's, and afterwards at 13 Stratford Place. This he did in the face of prolonged opposition. Notwithstanding, he enjoyed personal popularity, and amongst his acquaintances numbered such men as Dickens and Thackeray. Later he was appointed as medical adviser to the Duchess of Cambridge.

Of the first volume of Hahnemann's *Materia Medica Pura* Dr. Quin made a translation which was lost by fire at the printers. In 1844 this distinguished physician—whose distinction must have been the chief thorn in the side of his orthodox colleagues—founded the London Homœopathic Hospital.

England did not have her scourge of cholera

till 1853, some years after the rest of Europe. The outbreak happened just as the General Board of Health came into being under the first Public Health Act. This meant that for the first time carefully acquired statistics were available. In 1854 a report to the House of Commons gave the figures of death from cholera under orthodox treatment at 59.2 per cent., and under the homœopathic treatment at 16.4 per cent. In all 54,000 persons died.

Dr. McCloughlin, the Medical Inspector to the Government, who was not himself a homœopath, either by education, by practice, or by principle, stated that, of the cases treated in homœopathic hospitals, "all that I saw were true cases of Asiatic cholera, in the various stages of the diseases, and I saw several cases that did well under homœopathic treatment, which, I had no hesitation in saying, would have sunk under the other." The figures thus revealed soon after led Lord Ebury, during the passage of the Medical Act through the House of Lords, to win for homœopathy a continuance of its freedom in England by inserting a clause which prevented homœopathic physicians from being denied, on the ground of their beliefs, a place on the Medical Register then being set up.

It was no doubt as a result of the success which attended the adoption of Hahnemann's treatment that the Austrian Decree against homœopathy was withdrawn. There appears to have been a general extension of interest and a breakdown of official bias against it. In 1833 Dr. Baumann of Lahr, in Baden, wrote to Dr. Hahnemann of his method of healing thus:

> "It is making splendid progress in Baden, Alsace, and Switzerland, in spite of all the opposition put forth by its enemies. . . . The Homœopathic Society of Baden was founded under the chairmanship of Geheimer Hofrat Dr. Kramer, and I shall have the honour and pleasure to appear at Köthen as their delegate."

To his old acquaintance Counsellor Becker in Gotha, Hahnemann was also able to write in the year 1832: "You can hardly imagine how rapidly homœopathy is gaining in dear (I wish I could say peaceful) France."

Some time after von Brunnow wrote to the doctor from Dresden:

> "During recent years homœopathy has made still greater progress. How glad you must be, that even in the United States of North America a Society has been formed which bears your name, and which has for its object the propagation of your doctrine. The events in France also deserve the greatest consideration. . . . In Germany, at least in one State, Hessen-Darmstadt, self-dispensing has been accorded unhindered to homœopathic physicians. In Russia the practice of homœopathy has been allowed throughout the realm by a Ukase, and provision has been made for the erection of pure homœopathic chemist shops."

INTERNATIONAL DEVELOPMENTS

Despite large disappointments in many directions we can picture with what intense feelings of happiness the doctor must have opened his letters at this time, knowing that into countless stricken homes in various lands he had been able to introduce a medicine of peculiar virtues in meeting the scourge. Whether busy amongst his papers, receiving patients or guests, winding his several clocks on the mantelpiece, or sitting by the peat fire with his daughters, all these familiar occupations must by this have been rendered sweeter to the physician of seventy-eight years. With assurance he could observe: "The truth has already extended its rays too widely and shines too brightly to be eclipsed."

CHAPTER XIV

SECOND MARRIAGE AND CLOSING DAYS IN PARIS

Paris, 1832-1843

In 1829 Hahnemann wrote to Stapf:

"Your dear letter of September 3rd gave me the pleasantest expectation of seeing you soon here, and now your last letter, containing an absolute refusal to pay me a visit, has proportionately disappointed me. Do not serve me so! How do you know if next year, when the season is so far advanced that travelling becomes possible, I shall still be alive! That cannot be counted at all certain; and just consider for a moment how much we have still to talk over! . . . The prohibition of the homœopathic treatment of acute diseases in Russia is so abominable that it must be of the greatest advantage to us. Every educated person sees that it is a contrivance of the dominant allopathic sect, in order to divert the attention of the public from the remarkable superiority of homœopathic treatment of acute pleurisy. But what would such a strabismic government do if a homœopath were to cure a pneumonia or a pleurisy in a few hours? Would it condemn the homœopathic doctor to have his head cut off? Hardly in our time, not even in Russia."

Again, to the same friendly physician:

"Dear Friend and Colleague, fulfil your promise and make use of the beautiful sleigh road to give me the pleasure of a visit, for you cannot come to me often enough. But mind! you must bring friend Rummel with you. You will not wear that splendid ring? Is it not a real pleasure when without the slightest admixture of envy one can rejoice heartily and truly at the good fortune that has befallen a friend? . . . Therefore wear that ring when you visit a true friend, and confer a pleasure on him by so doing! But the letter that the Duke wrote to you is worth at least double the costly ring. The friend does not grudge you even that, but makes you heartily welcome to it, and is as much pleased as though the letter were written to himself. Now you know what you have to do in this case, and you will wear the ring in order to show it to a sympathising friend. Enclosed I return you Aegidi's letter. . . . I am happy to have been able to procure this good fortune for the excellent Aegidi, and in addition to the pay attached to the post he can freely and frankly practise homœopathy in a populous town under the protection of the ruler of the land, and may even prescribe his own medicines and dispense them unhindered to all his patients! If this is not a real piece of homœopathic good luck then I do not know what is..."

CLOSING DAYS IN PARIS

Whilst it may be true to say that the doctor's letters were almost entirely devoted to medical matters, nevertheless a sense of friendship for its own sake constantly crops up in them with unmistakable clearness.

A further letter also referring to an anticipated visit from Dr. Stapf, includes the information that the Baroness von Ende, a great patroness of literature, at that time living at Vevey, near Geneva, had been required by Sir Walter Scott, with whom she corresponded, to send him two copies of the fourth edition of the *Organon*, and that she had forwarded them to him in Edinburgh.

It would be interesting to know whether Sir Walter Scott, as a victim of blood-letting and other violent treatments then current, had heard of Hahnemann's vehement denunciations of them.

In one of his letters to Southey, Scott wrote:

"If I had not the strength of a team of horses I could never have fought through it, and through the heavy fire of medicinal artillery, scarce less exhausting—for bleeding, blistering, calomel, and ipecacuanha have gone on without intermission—while, during the agony of the spasms, laudanum became necessary in the most liberal doses, though inconsistent with the general treatment. I did not lose my senses, because I resolved to keep them, but I thought once or twice they would have gone overboard, top and top-gallants."

In January following this reference to the Baroness's letter an article on Homœopathy by Sir Daniel Sandford, a personal friend of Walter Scott, appeared in the Edinburgh Review. But it was not till December of that year that we find a postscript to a letter of Hahnemann's: "What about the Edinburgh Review?"

The article in question is remarkable for its humour, scepticism, and utter fairness. We can almost see the doctor reading it, while he reclined in the comfort of an armchair, and hear the outbreakings of gratified merriment as paragraph by paragraph made its appeal to him. Principal Albrecht has told us that it was Hahnemann's custom to share portions of his reading with members of his family. It would not be hard to believe that a considerable part if not the whole of this essay was thus read aloud.

The article also deals with some austerity with Hahnemann's critics.

"One party," says the writer, "accuses Hahnemann of false references; of misrepresentations of meaning when the references are correct; and, in short, of all the arts of unfair quotation. We are bound, however, to remark that, where we have taken the pains to verify his citations, we have not found Hahnemann guilty of the fraud thus imputed to his charge."

On the subject of small dosage the writer suggests: "Let us hear what the great homœopath has to say for himself, and what may be advanced from other sources in favour of this extraordinary part of this system." There follows a salient quotation from Hahnemann's writings, closing with the statement, "it is foolish to doubt the

CLOSING DAYS IN PARIS

possibility of that which in reality takes place, . . . since that which *actually happens* must at least be *possible*." Again, as regards the number of the cures under homœopathy, Sir Daniel Sandford states:

> "Such facts as we have above narrated—and the number might be considerably increased even from our own personal knowledge—are much insisted upon in support of the efficacy of the small doses. The number and the notoriety of the cures thus performed are, indeed, the main stumbling block to the antagonists of Hahnemann. Anything like an equal list of well-established instances of failure would be the best possible answer to Hahnemann's whole system. But these his opponents do not adduce. We have found nothing of the sort in any of the replies to the *Organon*, which we have perused. The case of Prince Schwartzenberg is the only example of failure brought forward. . . ."

"Listen to this," we can almost hear the doctor exclaiming to one or other of his family or circle of friends who had entered the room. And von Brunnow or Franz Hartmann, or it might be his daughter, would be given a seat to hear the paragraph out.

In 1834, Hahnemann, who had not visited Leipzig for thirteen years, went again to share in the June celebrations of the Homœopathic Hospital in that city. Dr. Lehmann, now Hahnemann's valued assistant in Köthen, together with Herr Isensee, Justice of the Peace, and the Hahnemann daughters, accompanied the doctor besides several others. Amongst these was Dr. Jahr of Gotha and the magistrate, Karl Rhost.

Hahnemann was now in his eightieth year. At the reception given to him he responded in German to Dr. Schweikert's address, which was in Latin, and afterwards dined with some of his friends and followers in his rooms at the hotel. Whether Rhost sang again the Latin song he had composed for the doctor's "Jubilee" is not mentioned. This was an adaptation of the well-known students' song *Gaudeamus*, in which the company are bidden to rejoice in being gathered together as the guests of Hahnemann.

It may be he composed another for this occasion, for although he was a lawyer managing his own estates of Pösigk and Cosa near Köthen, he lived, we are told, more for science, music and bright hospitality than for the plough.

In spite of the happiness of this event, in a city in which Hahnemann must have had many old connections, he returned to Köthen the following morning.

At no time was Hahnemann so satisfied with the hospital in Leipzig as when Dr. Schweikert had the direction of affairs. In an "Appeal to Homœopathic Physicians" we find the founder of homœopathy strongly recommending the institution to the support of those doctors who wished to see its survival, for the purpose of producing further good for science and mankind.

Dr. Schweikert was at the helm for two out of the first three years, but was disastrously followed in 1835 by a doctor, Fickel by name, who, on his resignation, admitted that he had entered the service of the hospital with the object of exposing homœopathy, and that he had even fabricated remarkable cases which had been believed by his colleagues to be true.

Of Hahnemann's great shrinking from any but attested cures we find a revelation in a letter written exactly ten years earlier:

> "Should our art once lose its attribute of the most conscientious exactness," he wrote to Stapf, "which must happen if the *dei minorum gentium* seek to push themselves into notoriety by their so-called observations, then I tremble for the raising of our art out of the dust; then we shall lose all certainty, which is of great importance to us. Therefore, I beg you will keep out of your *Archiv* all superficial observations of pretended successful treatment. Admit only truthful, accurate records of cases from the practice of accredited homœopaths; these must be models of good homœopathic art."

If Hahnemann's biographers are agreed that he was on occasions intensely intolerant, they must also recognise that this was mainly due to the fine degree in which he aspired to a realisation of perfection. The narrowness of his opportunities for clinical demonstration also, no doubt, contributed to his eagerness that all individual following of his method should be unfeigned. Haehl recognises this from another angle when he says that the severe harshness observed towards himself and towards others was in Hahnemann closely related to his restless creative impulse. None, indeed, are so restless as those whose movements are hampered by imposed restrictions. The accepted self-chosen limitations of the artist are another matter. Hahnemann felt, too, the impossibility of even attempting to combine things which in their very nature were diametrically opposed. To the great and revered physician, Hufeland, he wrote:

"But you, my dearest friend! endowed with the mild spirit of a Melanchthon, that would fain unite all opposing parties, bear with me,—since illusion will not amalgamate with truth,—bear with the pure-minded seeker after truth, who is inflexible in his convictions, incorruptible by the false doctrines and illusions of systems, even though you may not venture to take a bold glance into the reddening dawn, that must inevitably usher in the long-wished for day."

Soon after the visit to Leipzig an event occurred which was to translate Hahnemann into an entirely different sphere of home life and medical activity. A comparatively young French woman, Mademoiselle Melanie D'Hervilly, visited Köthen. It seems clear that her desire to see the Saxon doctor whose fame had reached her, was at least as strong as her wish to consult him. In a memoir in her own hand she describes herself as having been interested in medical matters from childhood, though her training later was as a painter.

At the time that Mademoiselle D'Hervilly came to Köthen the predilection for medicine was in the ascendency, and before long, though less than half his years, without hesitation she entered into a marriage based upon a mutual enthusiasm for the new art of healing.

The marriage took place on January 18th, 1835, but it was not immediately known even to some of his nearest friends. To these Hahnemann subsequently wrote with unqualified praise of his second wife Melanie. To Bönninghausen he described her as "a distinguished and excellent lady from Paris, handsome and tall and 32 years of age," adding, "I am separated from my last two daughters by walls alone. I have bought a house for them next to mine and furnished it for their own particular use; it is accessible to mine through the yard. . . . So far, I am very happy in my new arrangement, to attain which I had to overcome many difficulties."

From varied quarters letters of congratulation balanced the criticism with which this step was met. One of these was from Fischer in Meissen, a friend of Hahnemann's youth, a fact which again hints at Hahnemann's capacity for an enduring friendship.

One cause for perplexity seems to have lain in the fact that the French stranger had travelled to Köthen dressed as a man. Haehl comments that Goethe repeatedly allowed his most characteristic and attractive girl figures to appear in men's clothes. We know also that many characters in the literature of various lands had adopted the same rôle, notably in the ballad

Elise, the Flower of Serving Men. Being a woman of education it is quite likely that this unexpected intruder into the domestic circle at Köthen had read of these.

That Mademoiselle D'Hervilly was endowed with both poetic and philanthropic sentiments we know, for Hahnemann refers to a poem of hers written in earlier years, "l'Hirondelle d'Athènes," by means of which a considerable sum of money was obtained for the oppressed Greeks at the time. He refers also to an oil painting of himself by her, painted in Köthen, and therefore in the early months of their marriage. The trouble for which this patient had sought relief had been one which had, previous to her cure, prevented her from painting for three years.

Before long a project was conceived by the newly married pair to visit Paris together. This visit led to a permanent settlement in that city. Of this, Dr. Süss Hahnemann, a grandson living in London, wrote:

"Hahnemann had scarcely arrived in Paris when, through the influence of his young wife with King Louis Philippe, he received from the Minister Guizot the permission to practise, a concession which the Medical Faculty of Paris had refused. We suddenly find the old gentleman, who only shortly before that had expressed the earnest wish, and even written it down in his will, to retire from medical practice, surrounded by a widely-spread clientèle. In order to be able to practise

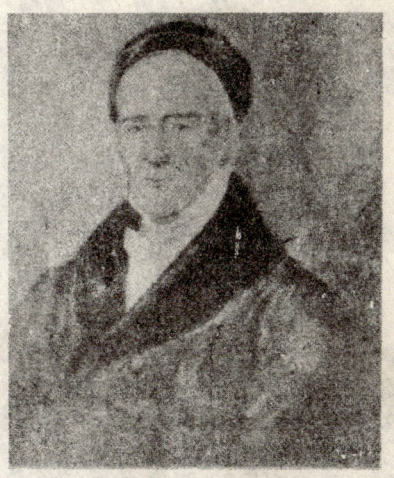

HAHNEMANN IN 1835, AFTER A PAINTING BY HIS SECOND WIFE

Faces page 262

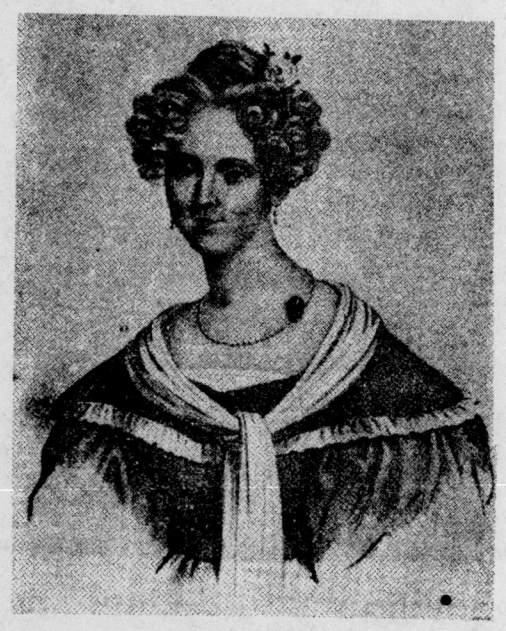

MADAME MELANIE, HAHNEMANN'S SECOND WIFE

Faces page 263

CLOSING DAYS IN PARIS

usefully he asked for the patients' records which he had already handed over to his daughter, with the most sincere promise that these volumes should be returned to his daughter after his death. With the sad foreboding that this treasure would never be seen by her again, his daughter Louise sent his manuscripts to Paris."

Nor were the daughter's fears unfounded. Had the adoption of man's attire been the only defect in the new Madame Hahnemann, Hahnemann's admirers would have found fairness to her less difficult. The most serious fault which they had to put against her was that for many years after Hahnemann's death, and even after her own, Melanie Hahnemann rendered it impossible for posterity to obtain access to Hahnemann's papers, including these most valuable records of cases. The eventual acquisition of these by the late Dr. Haehl in recent years led at length to the possibility of producing a more complete biography.

As homœopathy had for some time been practised in France, Madame Hahnemann's countrymen were able to give the founder of homœopathy an appreciation based on a very considerable acquaintance with his methods. A great ovation was arranged in the French capital. To the welcome accorded to him Hahnemann on the occasion made a sustained reply. It concluded warmly:

"Whilst exhorting the members of the Paris Society to unremitting and increased study,

I would like them to consider, as well as you all, gentlemen, that when we are dealing with a science which is concerned with the saving of life, it is *a crime to neglect its study*. . . And you, young men of France, who have not yet attained to the old errors, and are seeking for the truth in wakeful nights of work, come to me, because I bring you the truth you have long sought after, this sublime revelation of an eternal law of nature. I appeal to facts in trying to convince you; do not try to repudiate them until a conscientious and complete study assures you of success; then you, like me, will bless Providence for that immeasurable good, which has been allowed to descend upon the earth by my insignificant efforts, because I was only a feeble instrument of that Power before whom everything should remain humble."

Do we not catch in this the same vigorous enthusiasm which characterised his "Oratio," delivered before his masters and fellow-scholars on saying farewell to the Prince's School?

Nothing perhaps so clearly indicates the survival of the spirit of youth as a confident appeal from one full of years to the rising generation. As late as 1840 we catch the same note, only now with a strain of disappointment in it. This was in a passage addressed to his old friend Bönninghausen:

"Does not the medical youth of your district desire to become happy? But here, too, such conversions are rare, God pity them! If I do not notice an extraordinary desire for truth, I discourage them by pointing out to them the great difficulties entailed in learning thoroughly and practising our art. Many are deterred by it. But if they still remain firm in their intention, then I give them a helping hand, and all is well. They must also possess a kindness of heart and, if they have sufficient of that, they will not be lacking in gratitude towards their teacher and the divine art. When I have a safe opportunity through someone travelling, I will send you a good copper-etching of myself and something similar. We are both well and happy, in spite of all the burden of work, and love one another like good children."

We are reminded by this letter of the different ways in which, some years before, Hahnemann had responded to the unreliable seeker Robbi and the trustworthy disciple Constantine Hering. It was written only a few months after the celebration of the sixtieth jubilee of his doctorate, which was kept in Hahnemann's mansion in the Rue de Milan. From almost all the nations of Europe he received congratulations, some by letter, but most of them through representatives.

On his eighty-sixth birthday a further tribute reached him which, perhaps, more than equalled all others by reason of its tender associations with the years of his childhood. From the Town Council of Meissen he received a communication making him an "Ehrenbürger"—"honorary citizen," or, as we should say, his native town gave to him the "freedom of the City." In acknowledging this recognition of his life-work, Hahnemann wrote to the Magistrate at Meissen: "All that I have hitherto done for the welfare of the noble race of man, I regard only as a duty and a debt. May God bless Meissen and her trusty citizens!"

Speaking of Meissen's heritage in her sons when the city celebrated its own 1,000 years of existence, Dr. Preuss, then Latin master of the Prince's School, observed that the native of Meissen has every right to be proud of his great citizens of the past, "of Ludwig Richter and his charming deeply-felt pictures, of Böttger and Kändler, inventors of the exquisite china now so highly prized." "But," he adds, "pride is mingled with a deep and solemn reverence, when he is reminded of Dr. Samuel Hahnemann, the man who brought to suffering mankind new methods of healing disease."

Through the Paris period we find frequent affectionate letters from the father to his daughters with messages to his valued assistant Hofrat Lehmann, into whose care he had resigned his practice in Köthen.

"Dear Children," he wrote in one of these, "we thank you for your wishes as well as for the copy of the little songs with music, which are to brighten our hours of leisure and remind us of you. Take courage! Soon your wish to visit us in Paris may be fulfilled, as railways are progressing everywhere in Germany, and are already extending to Frankfort-on-Main, and also similarly in France up to the Rhine. Therefore remain in peace and live in hope as we do."

In a letter addressed to a doctor in Gotha we read of an informal gathering of lay homœopaths and homœopathic physicians passing through Paris held at his house each Monday for discussion.

Besides correspondence with Hering in America, Bönninghausen, Stapf, von Brunnow and others, we find more than one letter to Councillor von Gersdorff of Eisenach, which may serve us as a mirror to the home life and professional activities in Paris. We will quote from two together:

"Dearest friend and beloved Godfather, after our departure from Eisenach, where I and my dear Melanie had the pleasure of seeing you before saying good-bye, we arrived safely in Paris after short day stages on the 21st of June, at the house hitherto occupied by my wife. We were so well that even on the second day we were able to attend an excellent opera. As the first residence in the middle of the city did not seem suitable for the health of us both, we eagerly sought and found an excellent house which could not be surpassed for its advantages by any other house in the whole of great Paris. The windows of our servants' rooms look on to the street; our rooms (on the first floor), however, look out upon our garden which is well laid out and has an exit into the great garden of the

Luxembourg, providing a walk of half-an-hour in the purest country air to all who are fond of walking. On this side we live as if we were in the country, surrounded by most beautiful scenery, and are away from all noise, a thing which makes living in a city so unpleasant; yet on the other side we are actually in Paris, and the patients from Paris have easy access to me (also by carriage), as they are chiefly from the higher and highest classes. But I also give my help with pleasure to the poorest, for my excellent wife lends me a most helping hand, as she is a warm friend to our science. . . .

"Our consultations begin at 10 a.m. and last until 5 or 6 p.m. Every patient who can drive or walk is obliged to come to me, and I make no exceptions even for the most distinguished personages. Only those who are unable to walk or are bedridden receive a visit from us in the evening, whether they are rich or poor, unless it be urgently necessary to see them earlier in the day. Our horses are fleet and our carriage light. On those evenings when there are no patients to be seen we frequent the best theatres (among which the Italian theatre, the big Opera, and the Théâtre Français are the most prominent) or attend good concerts."

The latter part of this summary of daily occurrences belongs to a date at which Hahnemann had removed to the Rue de Milan, and is followed by the words:

"We live alone in a small mansion; we have a garden, and the air is very pure. Our servants are good: the cooking is of the best without being luxurious. I think that I shall be able to attain the object of my life here, which is to procure for our divine science, in this great capital of one and a half million inhabitants, recognition, confidence, and facilities. Jahr is living here now and is publishing the third edition of his *Repertory* in French. Kind regards to you, my dear friend, and to your beautiful family. Accept also the good wishes of my incomparable wife, and those of your Samuel Hahnemann."

There are incidents in his life in Paris that show Hahnemann unchanged in all but certain outward customs. One of these, told in after years when a man by the one concerned, John Young, may be given. At the age of twelve, in the period of Hahnemann's life at which we have arrived, Young had been brought by a wealthy benefactor from Scotland to see the famous Saxon physician. The boy had been ill for two years and the doctors had abandoned hope in his case.

"On the second day," he says, "after my arrival in Paris, Hahnemann visited me in my compartment, and his examination lasted roughly an hour and a half. I had to remain in bed and Hahnemann examined me minutely as no other doctor had done. . . . Then he declared that he now knew that I had come to him in time, and that he would be able to

I sought truth earnestly
and found it.

Rasch gesellschaft. Sasen losse;
Morgens ist nicht heut,
Keine Stunde laß entschlüpfe!
Selzig ist die Zeit.

Les plus inestimables trésors
sont une conscience irréprochable
et une bonne santé; l'amour
de Dieu et l'étude de soi-même
donne l'une, l'Homöopathie donne
l'autre

Paris, 12 Mars
1843

Samuel Hahnemann.

HAHNEMANN'S WRITING IN HIS EIGHTY-EIGHTH YEAR (see page 63).

cure me. I remember that his face had a luminous expression. He gave me the impression, I might almost say of a divine being, because there was something spiritual in his appearance. Without a doubt he was a good man, because I was told that he frequently said to his patients that he was doing his best, but he was only an instrument; 'God would have to give His blessing.'"

Yet even Hahnemann's prolonged and fruitful labours had to have an end. Soon after his eighty-eighth birthday, on which the doctor was in excellent health and spirits, he became affected with a bronchial trouble, to which he had been prone in the spring for a number of years. This time the illness was more acute and protracted. It lasted roughly for ten weeks and the doctor, who, until towards the end, prescribed for himself, appears to have known from the commencement that his days were drawing to a close. At times there were distressing attacks, due to increasing oppression. During one of these his wife expressed the thought that as he had relieved so many others and had suffered so many hardships in his arduous life, Providence surely owed to him exemption from all suffering.

"To me, why to me?" replied Hahnemann. "Everyone in this world works according to the gifts and powers which he has received from Providence, and *more* or *less* are words used only before the judgment seat of man, not before that of Providence. Providence owes nothing to me. I owe much to Providence. Yes, everything.

We know that for many years Hahnemann had philosophically faced the fact that death awaited him at the end of his journey. As far back as 1816 he had written in an already quoted letter on the birth of a child to Stapf:

> "In such a way I created for myself, during those heartrending hours, an inner life, such as we need for eternal survival and for our advent into the land of perfection. It is in vain that we hide from ourselves the fact that it is only for this end that we exist; we are led towards this exalted goal and nothing can hinder us. How quickly the first 30 years of your life vanished! Do you think that the 30 years that are now to come will not flee as quickly? Then you will be as close to the exit of this earthly school of preparation as the man who is writing this to you, and who has only a few years left to count among mortals, when he will cast off this earthly form pertaining to corruption, to enter calmly and cheerfully into the reign of the All-loving, the reign of truth, vision, and peace. Do not let us fall into any errors of calculation. A year has only twelve months. Only a small space is left before our goal is reached. Already the last hour, the last minute, of the passing to the Father of moral purity and virtue is vividly before my eyes, when I shall hardly be able to point upwards with my cold hand—and then the last moment. Simple,

joyful, and welcome is this moment to him who has striven to render himself worthy of it."

At five o'clock in the morning on July 2nd, 1843, Hahnemann died. Dr. Jahr, "the faithful scholar of the Köthen days," immediately visited the house.

Dr. Croserio, physician to the Sardinian Embassy in Paris, wrote of Hahnemann's last hours to another friend and colleague of the doctor's:

"How much equanimity, patience, and imperturbable goodness he exhibited! . . . he calmly made his final arrangements, and embraced each of his friends with tenderness, such as belongs to a final adieu, but with steady equanimity. His face expressed an ineffable calm. Death could not detract from the angelic goodness that belonged to the expression of his features."

Contrary to all that might have been expected of the distinction-loving Parisian, Madame Hahnemann, after having her husband's body embalmed, arranged for an almost secret funeral in the early hours of the morning of July 11th.

"We walked behind the hearse," wrote his grandson, Dr. Süss Hahnemann, "a very poor looking procession, to Montmartre. . . . It was an old vault built of brick which already contained two other coffins. . . . The immortal Founder of Homœopathy was buried like the poorest of the poor, only his wife, his daughter, myself, and Dr. Lethière being the mourners."

The comment follows that Hahnemann's wish to have the words "Non inutilis vixi—I have not lived in vain" engraved on his tomb was still unfulfilled twenty years afterwards.

But the followers of Christian Samuel Hahnemann of a later generation were not content to allow this forlorn grave in the cemetery of Montmartre to be their Master's last resting place, even though it might be argued that the body is but dust and it is the spirit that counts. In the year 1898 a reburial was sanctioned by the authorities in Paris and the doctor's remains were conveyed to the cemetery of Père Lachaise. To this ceremony representatives of the medical profession of France, Germany, Belgium, England, Italy, Russia, Spain, and the United States came. The inscription chosen by himself was also now accorded him with full recognition of its appropriateness: *Non inutilis vixi*.

"Here," writes Dr. Haehl, "Hahnemann rests, not far from the graves of the composers Rossini, Auber, and Donizetti. Near by lies the poet Racine and the latter's great contemporary, Molière. A fox on a grave marks the resting place of La Fontaine, the fable writer. Then comes science with the physicist and chemist, Gay-Lussac, the physicist and astronomer, Arago, and Gall, the founder of phrenology. Finally, in the same area are the representatives of war, the field-marshals of the first French Empire, Ney and Davoust.

Thus the grave of the German master of therapy lies in the Paris cemetery in the midst of France's famous dead, as one who worked, investigated, and fought in the service and for the good of all mankind."

Well may we ask, what has posterity done with the fruits of this man's labours—with his safer, surer, and more sensitive use of the healing virtues which often lie hidden in the deadliest poisons in the armoury of medicine? Or more pertinently, we may enquire what is being done in our own days to test his contribution to the healing art, with its claim to the discovery of a trustworthy law of operation upon which the physician can rely, to guide him in the selection of his remedies. Have those in charge of the general, fever, and mental hospitals, the sanatoriums and other public institutions made adequate trial to prove or disprove the findings of Hahnemann's tireless laboratory and clinical investigations? If there be anything beneficent in homœopathy, has this been made available for all, or are there blessings in its method which are still only enjoyed by a few, whilst the larger family of mankind are deprived of them?

"Let us now praise famous men," an ancient writer exclaims. And truly, since the influence of this man's work has reached to all parts of the world, we shall do well at least to know in what his greatness lay. Yet we can well doubt whether a man such as Christian Samuel Hahnemann can be praised except in the pursuit of his healing method. "The physician has no higher aim than to make sick folk well," he wrote—no other purpose than their restoration to health, which Flinders Petrie has described as "the marvellous joy of bodily recovery." "We find," as he continues with penetration, "the sense of praise and rejoicing in a new liberty of the soul to be a constant feature, where the poise of forces has been attained." Such a "sense of praise" is the only praise that this Saxon doctor would have coveted. It is the only living praise that posterity can give.

BIBLIOGRAPHY

Note.—The list below includes the more important of the works mentioned or quoted in the text, together with the principal authorities used by the writer.

WRITINGS OF C. F. S. HAHNEMANN

1775 *The Oratio:* On the Wonderful Construction of the Human Hand. (Printed in Dr. Preuss' work mentioned below.)

1782 Essays (in Krebs' *Medical Observations*).

1786 *On Poisoning by Arsenic: Its Treatment and Forensic Detection.*

1788 *On the Wine Test for Iron and Lead.*

1790 *Complete Directions for the Preparation of Mercurius Solubilis.*

1791 *Autobiography.* (Printed in Haehl's *Hahnemann: His Life and Work.*)

1793-99 *The Apothecaries' Lexicon.*

1796 *Description of Klockenbring during his Insanity.*

1805 *Fragmenta de viribus medicamentorum positivis, sive in sano corpore humano observatis.*

1810 *Organon of the Rational Art of Healing.* Trans. (1st ed.) by C. E. Wheeler, M.D., 1913. Also (5th ed.) by R. E. Dudgeon, M.D., 1849 (out of print).

1811–21 *Materia Medica Pura.* Trans. by R. E. Dudgeon, M.D., 1880.

1828 *Chronic Diseases.* Trans. by G. M. Scott, M.D., 1842.

1829 *Lesser Writings:* including essays in the *Friend of Health* I (1792) and II (1795). Trans. by R. E Dudgeon, M.D., 1851:

"On the Satisfaction of our Animal Requirements."

"On a New Principle for Ascertaining the Curative Power of Drugs" (1796).

"Are the Obstacles to Certainty and Simplicity in Practical Medicine Insurmountable?" (1797).

"Dietetic Conversation."

"View of Professional Liberality at the Beginning of the Nineteenth Century" (1801).

"Cure and Prevention of Scarlet Fever" (1801).

"Æsculapius in the Balance" (1805).

"Things that Spoil the Air."

"Socrates and Physon: on the Worth of Outward Show."

"The Medicine of Experience" (1806).

"The Prevention of Epidemics in General, especially in Towns."

"Protection against Infection in Epidemic Diseases."

BIBLIOGRAPHY

"Plans for Eradicating a Malignant Fever."

"On Making the Body Hardy."

"On the Choice of a Family Physician."

"On the Great Necessity of a Regeneration of Medicine: Extract from a Letter to a Physician of high standing [Hufeland]" (1808).

"Dissertation on the Helleborism of the Ancients" (1812).

[FOR OTHER WORKS, SEE OVER.]

OTHER WORKS

Albrecht, Franz, Principal. *Hahnemann's Leben und Wirken.* Leipzig (2nd ed.), 1875.

Allbutt, T. Clifford, M.D. *A System of Medicine by Many Writers.* (Vol. I.) London and New York, 1896.

Barker, W. Neish, M.D. *Hahnemann the Pioneer.* London, 1922.

Bier, August, Prof., Dr. med. *What shall be our Attitude to Homœopathy?* Munich. Trans. by P. J. R. Schmahl, M.D. Philadelphia (4th ed.) 1925.

Bönninghausen, Carl von. *Lesser Writings.* Trans. by Prof. L. H. Tafel. Philadelphia, 1908.

Bradford, Thomas Lindsey, M.D. *The Life and Letters of Dr. Samuel Hahnemann.* Philadelphia, 1895.

Braun, Lily. *Im Schatten der Titanen.* Brunswick, 1908.

Brunnow, Ernst von. *A Glance at Hahnemann and Homœopathy.* Leipzig, 1844. Trans. by J. Norton, 1845.

Burnett, J. C., M.D. *Ecce Medicus.* London, 1881.

Clarke, John H., M.D. *Dictionary of Materia Medica.* London, 1900.

BIBLIOGRAPHY

Garrison, Fielding H., M.D. *An Introduction to the History of Medicine*. Philadelphia and London (4th ed., revised and enlarged), 1929.

Haehl, Richard, M.D. *Samuel Hahnemann, His Life and Work*. Leipzig, 1922. Trans. by M. L. Wheeler and W. H. R. Grundy, B.A., London, 1931.

Haggard, H. W. *Devils, Drugs and Doctors*. London, 1929.

Hufeland, C. Wilhelm von, Prof. Dr. med. *Die Prophylactische Wirkung der Belladonna*. 1825.

Lewin, L., Prof., Dr. med. *Die Nebenwirkungen der Arzneimittel*. Berlin, 1899.

Meldola, Raphael, Prof., F.R.S. *Chemistry*. Revised by Prof. Alexander. Finlay. London, 1928.

Nixon, J. A., Prof., M.D. *The Debt of Medicine to the Fine Arts*. Bristol, 1923.

Preuss, Erich, Dr. phil. *Der Zwanzigjähriger Hahnemann (The Oratio)*. (Dr. Willmar Schwabe.) Leipzig, 1930.

Preuss, Erich, Dr. phil. Three articles in the *Leipziger Populäre Zeitschrift für Homöopathie*. (Dr. Willmar Schwabe.) Leipzig, June, 1929; February, 1930; December, 1931.

Sandford, Daniel, Sir. Article in *Edinburgh Review*. January, 1830.

Simpson, James Y., Sir. *Homœopathy*. Edinburgh (3rd ed.), 1853.

BIBLIOGRAPHY

Singer, Charles, M.D. *A Short History of Medicine.* Oxford, 1928.

Thompson, C. J. S. *The Mystery of the Art of the Apothecary.* London, 1929.

Wheeler, C. E., M.D. *The Case for Homœopathy* (British Homœopathic Association, Incor.) London (2nd ed.), 1923.

Wheeler, C. E., M.D. *Knaves or Fools.* London, 1908.

INDEX

Note.—The reader is referred to the Table of Contents (pp. 9-11) for Hahnemann's places of residence, and to the Bibliography for descriptions of the works both of Hahnemann and of the authors included in this Index.

Aegidi, Karl, 222 f., 240 f., 254; *and* illustration (224)
Ague (malaria), 76 ff.
Albrecht, Principal, *quoted*, 21, 177, 217, 235, 280
Allbutt, T. C., *quoted*, 128, 280
Amblyopia, 152
America, Homœopathy in. *See* United States
Anhalt-Köthen, Dukes of, 208 f., 219 f., 242
Apothecaries—
　Friendly relations with, 165, 207 f., 212 f.
　Guilds of, 163 ff.
　Opposition of, 199 ff. Status of, 50 f.
"Arcanists," 54-55
Aristotle, 33, 128, 191
Æsculapius in the Balance, chap. ix, 162 ff., 278
Apothecaries' Lexicon, 106 f., 213
Arndt-Schulz Law, preface, 145, 153
Arsenic, Poisoning by, 64, 72, 141, 277
Art, Influence of, 17, 29, 37, 52, 61, 99, 167
Austria, Homœopathy in, 198, 245, 249, Leopold II of, 81

Baden, Homœopathy in, 250
Barker, W. Neish, M.D., *quoted*, 151, 280
Bastanier, Ernst, Dr. med., 169
Becker, Councillor, 86, 90, 144, 159, 171, 250
Belladonna, 142 ff., 203
Bier, August, Dr. med., *quoted*, 138, 168, 280
Bloodletting. *See* Venesection
Bönninghausen, Carl von, 188 ff., 264, 267, 280
Botany, Hahnemann's interest in, 25, 29 f., 134-5, 234

INDEX

Böttger, Johann, 15 f., 266
Bradford, T. L., M.D., 8, 239, 280
Braun, Lily, 232, 280
Brukenthal, S. von, 42-3
Brunnow, E. von, *quoted*, 76, 195 ff., 200 f., 235, 250, 267, 280
Burnett, Dr. J. C., *quoted*, 68, 280

Camphor, 242, 245
Chamomilla, 188
Chemistry, Hahnemann's study of, 45, 49, 73, 106 f., 188
Cholera in Europe, 241 ff.; in England, 248 f.
Chronic Diseases, 222, 223 f., 278
Cinchona, 75; Experiment with, 76 ff.
Civic Responsibility, Hahnemann's sense of, 72, 107. *See also* Epidemics, Prison Reform, Town-Planning, Treatment of Insane
Clarke, Dr. J. H., *quoted*, 79, 168, 280
College, Cleveland Homœopathic Medical, U.S.A., 190
Colloids, 151
Cullen, 75 f., 79, 123

Demachy, 57, 106
Diet, Hahnemann's views on, 118
Drawing, Value of, 96
Dudgeon, Dr. R. E., 157, 277-8

Ebury, Lord, 249
Education, Hahnemann's views on, 30, 96, 116, 234
England, Homœopathy in, 247 ff.
Epidemics, 47-8, 70-1, 111, 278-9
Everest, Rev. T., 182

Fees, Hahnemann's views on, 89-91
Ferdinand of Anhalt, Duke, 208, 219, 222, 226 f.
France, Homœopathy in, 117, 238, 250, 263 f.
Freedom of the Press, Plea for, 169, 186
Freemasonry, 43, 206, 208
Friend of Health, Part I, 67 ff.; *Part II*, 107 ff., 278-9

Galen, 33, 35 f., 165
Garrison, Dr. F. H., *quoted*, 137, 281
Gay-Lussac, 127, 274
Gellert, 28, 169
Germ-life ("miasm"), Hahnemann's teaching *re*, 128, 243

INDEX

Goethe, 51, 80, 198, 202, 232, 261
Gold, Medicinal properties of, 150
Gross, Dr., 187-8, 240

Haehl, Dr. Richard, *quoted*, 7, 263, 281, *and passim*
Haggard, H. W., *quoted*, 137, 281
Hahnemann, Christian August, 16
  Christian Gottfried, 16 ff., 52 ff.
  Christoph, 17
  Henriette, 49, 52, 156-7, 183, 235 *and* illustration (160)
  Johanna, 17, 20
  Melanie, 260 ff. *and* illustration (263)
  Dr. Süss, 273
Hahnemann, Christian Samuel, Letters of, *quoted*, 72, 73, 90, 101-2, 104, 112, 122, 155, 158, 159, 169, 170 f., 186, 205-6, 218, 225, 228, 230, 232 ff., 247, 253 f., 259, 260, 264, 266, 267 ff., 272
Hahnemann's Portraits and Busts, 216-8, 226, 262, 265; *and see* illustrations
Hahnemann, Impressions of, 21, 32, 102-3, 179-81, 195-7, 237, 271, 273
Hartmann, Franz, Dr., 90, 178, 182-3, 187-8, 235
Häseler, Apothecary, 49, 52, 165
Hellebore, 136, 175 f.
Herbs, 30, 135, 162
Hering, Dr. C., 229-31, 267
Herrnhuters, Community of, 103, 207
Hippocrates, 33, 48, 73, 97 f., 115, 119
Hobhouse, Stephen, *quoted (but not always indicated by quote marks)*, 7, 13 f., 29 f., 31 ff., 37, 49 ff., 53 ff., 173, 181, 215
Holland, Homœopathy in, 244
Homœopathy, Birth of, 75 ff., 122, 130; Derivation of, 132, 146
  Chair of, 169
Hörold, Commissioner, 16
Hospital, First Homœopathic, 226-7, 257; First Children's Homœopathic, 223
Hufeland, C. W., Prof., 80, 122, 132 ff., 185, 203, 232, 243, 260, 279, 281

Insane, Treatment of, chapter v *passim;* 118, 155-6
Insect-life, Hahnemann's interest in, 24, 139, 218
Italy, Homœopathy in, 239, 247-8

INDEX

Jahr, Dr., 258, 269, 273

Kant, 104
Koch, 243

Lappe, Apothecary, 207 f.
Lavoisier, 59
Law of cure, 79, 125
Laymen, Hahnemann's attitude to, 162, 188, 191, 267, **268**
Lehmann, Dr., 221, 257, 266; *and see* illustration (209)
Lesser Writings, Hahnemann's, 168, 226, 228, 278; Bönninghausen's, 191, 280
Lewin, Prof. L., 78, 142, 281
Louis Philippe, King, 262
Lutze, Dr., 117, 215 f.

Marriage, Hahnemann's ideal of, 61, 69, 157-8, **233**
Materia Medica Pura, 14, 138, 225, 248, 278
McCloughlin, Dr., medical inspector, 249
Meissen, chapters i and ii, 51, 180 f.; Hahnemann "Ehrenbürger" of, 265-6
Meissen, Frauenkirche, 14, 181; Porcelain Factory, 15 ff., 53 f.; Prince's School, 14, 22, 27, 31 ff., 37 f., 169
Meldola, Prof. R., *quoted*, 15, 127, 152, 281
Metallurgy, 47
Monuments to Hahnemann, 17, 174, 215, 274; *and see* illustration (224)
Müller, Adam, Austrian Consul, 209 ff., 219, 239
Müller, Magister, 22, 24, 27 f.

Napoleon I, 170, 186
Napoleon III, 190
Nixon, Dr. J. A., *quoted*, 97, 281

Observation, Faculty of, 95 f., 188
Oratio, 31 ff.
Organon, 77, 92, 128, 167, 169, 184-5, 192, 257, 277

Palliatives, Hahnemann's attitude to, 129-30
Pappenheim, Countess von, 231
Paracelsus, 137-8
Pasteur, 243
Pathology, Hahnemann's valuation of, 122, 128
Philology, Hahnemann's love of, 58, 177
Pinel, 85, 95

INDEX

Plato, Influence of, 33, 35, 99, 104
Poisons, Hahnemann's view of, 64, 140-1
Politics, Hahnemann's interest in, 186, 226
Poor, Hahnemann's attitude to the, 70, f., 84, 90, 239, 268
Poverty, Hahnemann's attitude to, 48, 71, 108, 113
Potentisation, 145-6, 153
Poynton, Dr. A. B., *quoted*, 37
Preuss, Dr. Erich, *quoted*, 7, 21, 31, 37, 181, 266, 281
Prison Reform, 59-60
"Prover's Union," 187 f., 191-3
Psora, 223-4

Quarin, Dr., 40 ff., 123
Quin, Dr. F. F., 247-8

Religious Outlook, Hahnemann's, 32 ff., 40, 97, 103, 123-5, 139-40, 141-2, 158, 230-1, 233, 264, 271-3
Rousseau, Influence of, 67-8
Russia, Homœopathy in, 250, 253

Sandford, Sir Daniel, *quoted*, 256 f., 281
Saxony, Electors of, 27, 53 f.; August, 15-16; Moritz, 22
Scarlet Fever, Treatment of, *see* Belladonna
Schultz, Hugo, 153, 168
Schwabe, Dr. Willmar, Leipzig, 7, 281
Schwarzenberg, General Prince von, 198 ff., 202, 257
Scott, Sir Walter, 255 f.
Self-dispensing (and the 'preparing' of medicines), 164, 166-7, 199-201, 204, 206-7, 209-12, 254
Shrewsbury, Earl of, 247
Signatures, Doctrine of, 137 f.
Similars, Law of, 76, 78, 92, 130, 134, 136, 138, 142, 153
Simpson, Dr. James, *quoted*, 160, 281
Singer, Dr., *quoted*, 48, 95, 149, 282
Society, Hahnemann, U.S.A., 250
Society of Homœopathic Physicians, 227
Stapf, Dr., 183 f., 186, 187, 193, 228, 240, 253-5, 259, 267, 272; *and see* illustration (161)

Thompson, C. J. S., *quoted*, 75, 282
Town-planning, 116
Translating work, Hahnemann's, 39, 57, 61, 63, 67, 106, 162
Tuke, William, 85
Tyler, Margaret, Dr., *quoted*, 8, 193

INDEX

United States, Homœopathy in, 190, 229, 250. *See also* illustration (224)

Universities: Berlin (Chair of Homœopathy), 169; Erlangen, 44, 226; Heidelberg (introduction of microscopy and chemistry), 45; Leipzig, 38, 62, 174 f., 210

Veith, Father, 245-6
Venesection, 79 ff., 255

War, Hahnemann's views on, 141, 156, 187
Weir, Sir John, *quoted*, preface, 14, 153
Wheeler, C. E., M.D., *quoted*, 8, 64, 77, 168, 277, 282
Wine Test, Hahnemann's, 63-4

Youth Appeal to, 34, 264